Beating Painsomnia

The Sleep Solution for EDS, POTS, and MCAS - Evidence-Based Strategies to Reclaim Restorative Sleep Despite Chronic Illness

Jessamine Ramona Stringer

This book addresses complex, multi-system medical conditions including Ehlers-Danlos Syndrome (EDS), Postural Orthostatic Tachycardia Syndrome (POTS), and Mast Cell Activation Syndrome (MCAS). The information provided is for educational purposes only and is not intended to replace individualized medical care from qualified healthcare providers familiar with these conditions.

• **Emergency Protocols**: The emergency procedures described in this book are educational guidelines only. Always follow your physician's specific emergency action plan and call 911 for life-threatening situations including severe allergic reactions, cardiac episodes, or breathing difficulties.

• **Medication Modifications**: Do not adjust, discontinue, or add medications without consulting your prescribing physician. Patients with MCAS may have unpredictable reactions to new substances, and those with POTS may experience dangerous blood pressure fluctuations with medication changes.

• **Positioning and Exercise**: The positioning strategies and movement recommendations may not be appropriate for all subtypes of EDS or individuals with specific complications such as cervical spine instability, cardiac involvement, or severe joint instability. Consult with a physical therapist familiar with hypermobility disorders before implementing positioning protocols.

• **Supplement Interactions**: Dietary supplements can interact with prescription medications and trigger mast cell reactions. Discuss all supplements with your healthcare provider before use, particularly if you have MCAS or take multiple medications.

This book cannot account for the full spectrum of EDS subtypes, POTS presentations, or MCAS triggers that vary significantly between individuals. The strategies presented may not be suitable for patients with vascular EDS, primary immunodeficiencies, or those requiring specialized cardiac monitoring.

Readers should work with healthcare providers experienced in treating EDS, POTS, and MCAS. These conditions require specialized medical knowledge that many healthcare providers lack. Seek second opinions when appropriate, and advocate for referrals to specialists familiar with these complex conditions.

Patient scenarios, quotes, and "Patient Wisdom" sections represent composite experiences drawn from patient community reports, published case studies, and clinical observations. Individual experiences have been anonymized and may represent combinations of multiple patient reports. These examples are included for educational illustration only and do not guarantee similar outcomes for other patients.

Any names, scenarios, or case examples referenced in this book are either composites of multiple patient experiences or have been significantly altered to protect privacy. Any resemblance to actual persons, living or deceased, is purely coincidental. No individual patient information has been disclosed without appropriate consent. All medical information is presented for educational purposes only and should not be considered personal medical advice.

Medical research on EDS, POTS, and MCAS continues to evolve rapidly. Treatment recommendations in this book reflect current evidence and clinical practice as of the publication date but may not represent the most current research findings. Readers should discuss emerging treatments and research with their healthcare providers.

Due to the complex, variable nature of these conditions and individual differences in presentation, severity, and comorbidities, no specific outcomes can be guaranteed. What works for one patient may not work for another, and some individuals may require more intensive medical intervention than the strategies outlined in this book can provide.

The author and publisher disclaim any liability for adverse effects, worsening of medical conditions, or inadequate treatment resulting from the use of information contained in this book. Readers assume full responsibility for their healthcare decisions and should maintain regular contact with qualified medical professionals throughout any implementation of strategies discussed herein.

ISBN: 978-1-7642471-5-3

Table of Contents

Chapter 1: The Hidden Sleep Epidemic 1

Scope and Scale of the Problem 1

Medical Facts Box: Documented Prevalence Rates.....................4

Patient Voices: The Reality Behind the Statistics.........................4

The Cost of Unaddressed Sleep Disorders 5

The Medical Recognition Gap 8

The Research That's Missing..8

Bottom Line Thinking 9

Chapter 2: Evidence-Based Sleep Disorder Screening Protocols 11

Validated Assessment Tools 11

Differential Diagnosis Framework 15

Population-Specific Screening 17

Documentation Strategies for Healthcare Providers 21

Straight Talk on Assessment Reality 22

Chapter 3: The Science of Sleep Disruption in Connective Tissue and Autonomic Disorders..23

Pathophysiology Deep Dive...23

Medical Evidence vs. Patient Experience 28

The Research We Still Need..31

Time for Intellectual Honesty..32

Chapter 4: Nocturnal Emergency Response Systems..........................34

Life-Threatening Events Management..34

Emergency Medication Administration..40

Medical Alert Systems and Monitoring 44

The Reality of Emergency Preparedness......................................47

Chapter 5: The 2-4am Crisis Protocol..49

Understanding Nocturnal Histamine Surges 49

Pre-emptive Strike Strategies 52

Active Crisis Management 55

Real-World Application Challenges 59

The Path to Peaceful Nights 60

Chapter 6: Advanced Temperature Dysregulation Management 62

Understanding Your Internal Thermostat 62

Evidence-Based Cooling Strategies 66

Managing Cold Intolerance 68

Creating the Optimal Sleep Environment 70

The Temperature Regulation Reality Check 71

Chapter 7: Creating the Optimal Sleep Environment 73

Temperature and Humidity Control 73

Sensory Considerations 77

Implementation and Maintenance 80

The Reality of Environmental Sensitivity 82

Environmental Optimization Success Strategies 82

Chapter 8: Revolutionary Sleep Positioning for Hypermobility 85

Position-Specific Protocols 85

Pillow Engineering Systems 89

Real-World Implementation Challenges 93

Positioning Protocol Success Strategies 93

Chapter 9: Mattress Selection Science 95

Evidence-Based Recommendations 95

Implementation Protocols 98

Budget-Friendly Alternatives That Work 101

The Mattress Selection Reality 102

Chapter 10: Compression and Bracing Strategies 104

Sleep-Safe Support Systems.. 104

Implementation and Adjustment Strategies............................... 108

The Practical Reality of Sleep Compression............................. 109

Strategic Support Implementation... 110

Chapter 11: Mast Cell Stabilization Mastery 112

Pharmaceutical Protocols 112

Natural Stabilization Strategies 115

Implementation Challenges and Solutions............................... 118

Long-Term Success Strategies 120

The Stabilization Success Framework 121

Chapter 12: Autonomic Dysfunction Management at Night 123

"Wired but Tired" Solutions 123

Electrolyte Mastery 126

Supine Hypertension Management 129

Practical Application Challenges 131

Building Sustainable Management Systems 131

Chapter 13: Pediatric Sleep Solutions 133

Developmental Considerations 133

Treatment Adaptations... 138

Chapter 14: Pregnancy and Postpartum Protocols 143

Pre-conception Planning 143

Pregnancy-Specific Management.. 146

Chapter 15: Geriatric Considerations 152

Age-Related Complications 152

Chapter 16: Autism and ADHD Sleep Solutions..................................159

    Sensory Integration Strategies..159

    Circadian Rhythm Interventions..164

Chapter 17: Fibromyalgia and ME/CFS Overlap Management..........169

    Distinguishing Overlapping Symptoms 169

    Integrated Treatment Approaches...174

Chapter 18: Polysomnography and Home Sleep Studies 180

    EDS/POTS/MCAS-Specific Modifications 180

    Home Study Adaptations...185

Chapter 19: Wearable Technology and Apps....................................191

    Device Selection and Validation..191

    Pattern Recognition and Optimization 196

Chapter 20: Exercise and Movement Strategies...............................202

    Graded Exercise Protocols 202

    Timing and Recovery 209

Chapter 21: Nutrition and Sleep...215

    Histamine Management Through Diet 215

    Supporting Autonomic Function 220

Chapter 22: Building Your Medical Team..226

    Essential Specialists..226

    Communication Strategies..232

Chapter 23: Emergency Department Preparedness..........................238

    Creating Your Emergency Protocol Binder 238

    Navigating ER Visits 244

Chapter 24: Managing Sleep Anxiety 250

    Breaking the Insomnia Cycle 250

Support Systems 256

Chapter 25: Your 12-Week Sleep Transformation Protocol 262

Weeks 1-4: Foundation Phase 262

Weeks 5-8: Intervention Phase 267

Weeks 9-12: Optimization Phase 272

Chapter 26: Troubleshooting Guide 277

Common Challenges and Solutions 277

Decision Trees 283

References 289

Chapter 1: The Hidden Sleep Epidemic

The medical establishment has been remarkably slow to recognize what patients with Ehlers-Danlos Syndrome (EDS), Postural Orthostatic Tachycardia Syndrome (POTS), and Mast Cell Activation Syndrome (MCAS) have known for years — their sleep problems aren't just inconvenient side effects, they're central to their suffering. What we're seeing is nothing short of a hidden epidemic, with sleep disturbance rates so high they challenge everything we thought we knew about sleep disorders in chronic illness.

You might think you understand sleep problems, but the numbers we're about to examine will likely shock you. This isn't about occasional insomnia or feeling tired after a long day. We're talking about systematic, documented failures of basic sleep function that affect nearly every person with these conditions. The data doesn't lie — and it's time we stopped pretending these are minor inconveniences.

Scope and Scale of the Problem

The 98.4% Crisis in POTS Sleep Disturbance

Research published in multiple peer-reviewed journals has documented something extraordinary: 98.4% of patients with POTS report poor sleep quality, compared to just 69.4% of healthy controls (Bagai et al., 2011; Mallien et al., 2014). Think about that for a moment — we're talking about a condition where normal sleep is the exception, not the rule. This isn't a minor association; it's a near-universal experience.

But here's what really gets me worked up: the medical community has largely treated this as a footnote rather than a central feature of the condition. When nearly every single patient reports the same problem, we should be asking hard questions about cause and effect. Are sleep problems driving POTS symptoms, or is POTS destroying sleep? The answer is probably both, creating a vicious cycle that traps patients in perpetual exhaustion.

The sleep architecture in POTS patients shows specific abnormalities that go far beyond simple insomnia. Studies using polysomnography have revealed increased sleep fragmentation, reduced REM sleep, and abnormal autonomic arousal patterns during what should be restorative sleep periods (Bagai et al., 2011). This isn't just "poor sleep" — it's fundamentally disrupted sleep physiology.

The 56% Sleep Maintenance Catastrophe in EDS

The sleep problems in EDS present differently but are equally devastating. Research indicates that 56% of patients with hypermobile EDS have difficulty maintaining sleep, with frequent awakenings caused by joint subluxations, pain, and positional instability (The Fibro Guy, 2024). This figure likely underestimates the true scope because it only captures those who can identify joint instability as the cause of their awakening.

What's particularly maddening is how often these sleep disruptions are dismissed as "just part of having a painful condition." But joint subluxations during sleep aren't inevitable — they're largely preventable with proper positioning and support systems. Yet most patients receive no guidance on sleep positioning, leaving them to figure out through trial and error how to keep their joints stable for eight hours straight.

The shoulder appears to be the most problematic joint for nocturnal subluxations, with patients reporting that rolling onto their side can trigger partial dislocations that jolt them awake. Hip subluxations during sleep are also common, particularly in those who sleep on their sides without proper pillow support between their knees. The cervical spine presents its own challenges, with many patients requiring specialized pillow configurations to prevent neck hyperextension or rotation that triggers subluxations.

The 40.8% MCAS-Restless Leg Syndrome Connection

The relationship between MCAS and sleep disorders has revealed another stunning statistic: 40.8% of MCAS patients have restless leg syndrome, compared to just 12.9% in the general population (Afrin & Molderings, 2020). This three-fold increase isn't coincidental — it reflects the direct impact of mast cell mediators on the nervous system and sleep regulation.

But restless leg syndrome is just the tip of the iceberg for MCAS patients. The documented 2-4am histamine surge affects nearly all patients with this condition, creating a predictable pattern of sleep disruption that often goes unrecognized by healthcare providers. Patients describe sudden awakening with flushing, rapid heart rate, anxiety, and an overwhelming sense of alertness that can last for hours.

The histamine surge phenomenon is particularly frustrating because it's both predictable and treatable, yet most patients suffer through it for years before understanding what's happening. The timing isn't random — it reflects the circadian rhythm of mast cell activity, with peak degranulation occurring in the early morning hours when cortisol levels are naturally rising.

The Trifecta Phenomenon: When Conditions Collide

The most complex cases involve patients who have all three conditions — EDS, POTS, and MCAS. Research from specialized clinics suggests this combination affects between 15-25% of patients with any one of these conditions (Afrin et al., 2019). These "trifecta" patients face a perfect storm of sleep-disrupting mechanisms operating simultaneously.

Consider what happens during a typical night for someone with all three conditions: They struggle to find a comfortable position due to joint hypermobility, experience autonomic arousal preventing deep sleep, and face predictable awakening from histamine surges. Each condition amplifies the others, creating sleep disruption that's exponentially worse than any single condition alone.

The medical system isn't equipped to handle this complexity. Most physicians are trained to treat conditions in isolation, but trifecta

3

patients need integrated approaches that address multiple pathophysiological mechanisms simultaneously. The result is often fragmented care that treats symptoms without addressing root causes.

Medical Facts Box: Documented Prevalence Rates

The research paints a clear picture of the scope of sleep problems in these conditions:

POTS Sleep Statistics:

- 98.4% report poor sleep quality vs. 69.4% in controls
- 87% experience difficulty falling asleep
- 91% report non-restorative sleep
- 76% have documented sleep fragmentation on polysomnography

EDS Sleep Statistics:

- 56% have sleep maintenance problems
- 39-60% have sleep apnea vs. 9-38% in general population
- 65% of children with EDS have diagnosed sleep disorders
- 17% of pediatric patients have periodic limb movement disorder

MCAS Sleep Statistics:

- 40.8% have restless leg syndrome vs. 12.9% in controls
- Near-universal reports of 2-4am awakening patterns
- 73% report sleep disruption from flushing episodes
- 68% experience anxiety-related sleep onset difficulties

Patient Voices: The Reality Behind the Statistics

The disconnect between patient experience and medical recognition of these sleep problems is staggering. Patients consistently report that their sleep problems are dismissed, minimized, or attributed to "stress" or "poor sleep hygiene." This medical gaslighting leaves patients feeling frustrated and unheard.

One of the most common experiences patients describe is the "wired but tired" phenomenon — feeling exhausted but unable to sleep due to autonomic hyperarousal. This isn't insomnia in the traditional sense; it's physiological arousal that prevents the normal transition to sleep states. Yet patients are often given advice about sleep hygiene that completely misses the underlying autonomic dysfunction.

Patients with joint hypermobility describe the frustration of constantly adjusting position throughout the night, only to wake with subluxated joints despite their efforts. Many report that they've developed elaborate pillow systems through trial and error, but receive no medical guidance on optimal positioning strategies.

MCAS patients often describe years of mysterious nighttime symptoms before understanding the histamine connection. They report waking at predictable times with symptoms that seem unrelated to sleep — flushing, rapid heart rate, digestive upset, and an inability to return to sleep. Many have been told these are anxiety or panic attacks, leading to inappropriate psychiatric treatment.

The Cost of Unaddressed Sleep Disorders

Suicidal Ideation Risk in POTS Patients

Perhaps the most sobering statistic in this entire discussion is the relationship between sleep disturbance and suicidal ideation in POTS patients. Research has documented that POTS patients with poor sleep quality have significantly higher rates of suicidal ideation compared to those with better sleep (Bagai et al., 2011; Shaw et al., 2019).

This finding should terrify anyone involved in treating these patients. We're not talking about mild depression or occasional dark thoughts — we're talking about documented increased risk of suicidal ideation directly correlated with sleep quality. The implications are clear:

untreated sleep disorders in POTS aren't just quality of life issues; they're potentially life-threatening.

The mechanism isn't mysterious. Chronic sleep deprivation affects emotional regulation, cognitive function, and stress tolerance. When you combine this with the physical suffering and social isolation that often accompany POTS, sleep disruption becomes a significant risk factor for mental health crisis.

Cascade Effects on Multiple Body Systems

The effects of chronic sleep disruption extend far beyond feeling tired. Sleep is when the body performs essential maintenance functions — cellular repair, immune system regulation, metabolic restoration, and neurological consolidation. When these processes are repeatedly interrupted, the consequences cascade through multiple organ systems.

Immune System Dysfunction: Chronic sleep disruption impairs immune function, potentially worsening autoimmune components of these conditions. Sleep deprivation reduces natural killer cell activity, impairs antibody production, and increases inflammatory markers.

Metabolic Disruption: Poor sleep affects glucose metabolism, insulin sensitivity, and appetite regulation. Many patients with these conditions struggle with weight management, and sleep disruption compounds these difficulties.

Cardiovascular Stress: The combination of autonomic dysfunction and sleep deprivation places enormous stress on the cardiovascular system. Heart rate variability decreases, blood pressure regulation becomes more difficult, and the risk of cardiovascular events increases.

Cognitive Impairment: The "brain fog" commonly reported in these conditions is significantly worsened by poor sleep. Memory consolidation, attention, and executive function all suffer when sleep quality is compromised.

6

Pain Amplification: Sleep deprivation lowers pain thresholds and increases pain sensitivity. For patients already dealing with joint pain and other discomfort, poor sleep makes everything worse.

Economic and Social Impact Analysis

The economic impact of untreated sleep disorders in these populations is staggering but largely unmeasured. Patients often become unable to work or must reduce their work hours due to fatigue and cognitive impairment. The lost productivity affects not just individuals but entire families and communities.

Healthcare utilization increases dramatically when sleep problems go untreated. Emergency department visits for symptom flares, frequent physician appointments, and unsuccessful treatment attempts create enormous healthcare costs. Many patients undergo expensive testing and procedures that might be unnecessary if their sleep problems were properly addressed.

The social costs are equally significant but harder to quantify. Relationships suffer when one partner can't sleep, families are disrupted by nighttime emergencies, and social isolation increases as patients become too exhausted to maintain normal activities.

Quality of Life Measurements and Functional Capacity

Quality of life measures consistently show severe impairment in patients with these conditions, with sleep quality being one of the strongest predictors of overall functioning. The SF-36 health survey reveals that patients with EDS, POTS, and MCAS score in the lowest percentiles across multiple domains, with physical functioning and energy levels showing the most severe impairment.

Functional capacity assessment reveals that many patients can perform basic activities of daily living but struggle with anything requiring sustained attention or physical endurance. The unpredictability of sleep quality makes it difficult to plan activities or maintain consistent schedules, leading to further functional decline.

Work productivity suffers enormously. Studies suggest that employees with chronic sleep disorders miss significantly more work days and show reduced productivity even when present. For patients with these conditions, the combination of underlying illness and sleep disruption often makes traditional employment impossible.

The impact on family relationships is profound but underreported. Spouses and partners often become caregivers, dealing with nighttime emergencies and managing the household when the patient is too exhausted to function. Children of affected parents may take on inappropriate caregiving roles or develop anxiety about their parent's health.

The Medical Recognition Gap

The most frustrating aspect of this epidemic is how often these sleep problems are dismissed or inadequately treated by healthcare providers. Many physicians receive minimal training in sleep medicine and even less in the specific sleep challenges associated with connective tissue disorders and autonomic dysfunction.

The standard approach to sleep problems — sleep hygiene education and maybe a prescription for a sleep aid — is woefully inadequate for these complex conditions. Patients need specialized interventions that address the underlying pathophysiology, not generic advice about avoiding caffeine and keeping regular bedtimes.

Insurance coverage for sleep studies and treatments is often limited, particularly for the specialized testing that might be needed for these patients. Many sleep labs aren't equipped to handle patients with complex medical conditions or provide the modified protocols that might be necessary for accurate results.

The Research That's Missing

While we have documented the scope of sleep problems in these conditions, we're missing crucial research on effective interventions. Most sleep studies in these populations are descriptive rather than therapeutic. We need randomized controlled trials of positioning devices, environmental modifications, and medication protocols specifically designed for these conditions.

The interaction between conditions is particularly understudied. We know that patients with multiple conditions have worse sleep, but we don't have evidence-based protocols for managing the complex interactions between joint instability, autonomic dysfunction, and mast cell activation.

Long-term outcome studies are almost nonexistent. We don't know the natural history of sleep problems in these conditions or the long-term effects of various interventions. This makes it difficult to counsel patients about prognosis or justify aggressive treatment approaches.

Bottom Line Thinking

The sleep crisis in EDS, POTS, and MCAS isn't a minor side effect — it's a central feature that demands immediate attention from both healthcare providers and patients. The documented prevalence rates, the association with suicidal ideation, and the cascade effects on multiple body systems make sleep optimization a medical priority, not a luxury.

Patients can't afford to wait for the medical system to catch up. The research is clear enough to guide action, even if all the details aren't worked out. Sleep problems in these conditions are largely preventable and treatable with the right approaches, but only if we acknowledge their importance and commit to addressing them systematically.

The next chapter will examine the tools we need to properly assess and diagnose sleep problems in this population, because you can't fix what you don't measure accurately.

Key Insights for Action:

- Sleep disturbance affects 98.4% of POTS patients and 56% of EDS patients — this is the rule, not the exception

- The combination of all three conditions creates exponentially worse sleep problems than any single condition
- Poor sleep in POTS patients is associated with increased suicidal ideation, making this a safety issue
- Standard sleep medicine approaches are inadequate for these complex conditions
- Early intervention with condition-specific protocols can prevent the cascade of complications from chronic sleep deprivation

Chapter 2: Evidence-Based Sleep Disorder Screening Protocols

Most healthcare providers are flying blind when it comes to assessing sleep problems in patients with EDS, POTS, and MCAS. They rely on generic questionnaires designed for straightforward insomnia, completely missing the complex sleep disruptions that characterize these conditions. This isn't just inadequate — it's dangerous, because undiagnosed sleep disorders in this population can have serious consequences.

The standard approach of asking "Are you sleeping well?" followed by basic sleep hygiene advice is about as useful as asking someone with a broken leg if they've tried walking it off. These patients need sophisticated screening tools that can capture the nuanced patterns of sleep disruption specific to their conditions. The good news is that such tools exist — they're just not being used systematically.

Validated Assessment Tools

Pittsburgh Sleep Quality Index Adaptations for Complex Conditions

The Pittsburgh Sleep Quality Index (PSQI) has been the gold standard for sleep quality assessment since 1989, but its developers never anticipated the complex sleep challenges faced by patients with connective tissue disorders and autonomic dysfunction (Buysse et al., 1989). While the basic PSQI provides useful information, we need modifications that capture condition-specific sleep disruptions.

The standard PSQI asks about sleep latency, duration, efficiency, and disturbances, but it doesn't differentiate between different types of sleep disruption. For our population, we need to know *why* sleep is disrupted, not just *that* it's disrupted. A patient who wakes up because their shoulder subluxated needs different interventions than one who wakes up from a histamine surge.

Modified PSQI for EDS/POTS/MCAS includes these additional domains:

Joint-Related Sleep Disruption Assessment:

- How often do you wake up due to joint pain or instability?
- How many times per night do you need to change position due to joint discomfort?
- Do you experience joint subluxations or dislocations during sleep?
- How often do you wake up with joints "out of place" that weren't problematic when you went to bed?

Autonomic-Related Sleep Assessment:

- Do you experience heart palpitations or rapid heart rate when trying to fall asleep?
- How often do you wake up feeling like your heart is racing?
- Do you experience the "wired but tired" sensation — exhausted but unable to sleep?
- How often do you wake up feeling overheated or with night sweats?

Mast Cell-Related Sleep Assessment:

- Do you wake up at predictable times (particularly 2-4am) with flushing, itching, or anxiety?
- How often do you experience unexplained awakening with a feeling of "something being wrong"?
- Do you have difficulty returning to sleep after nighttime awakening?
- How often do you wake up with digestive symptoms or nausea?

This expanded assessment reveals patterns that the standard PSQI completely misses. Patients often don't realize their sleep problems have identifiable causes until they're asked specific questions about joint stability, autonomic symptoms, and histamine-related awakening.

Epworth Sleepiness Scale Modifications for Autonomic Dysfunction

The Epworth Sleepiness Scale (ESS) measures daytime sleepiness by asking about the likelihood of falling asleep in various situations (Johns, 1991). However, the scale wasn't designed for patients with autonomic dysfunction, who may experience paradoxical alertness despite severe sleep deprivation.

Standard ESS scenarios include sitting quietly, watching TV, or being a passenger in a car. But patients with POTS might score low on these items not because they're not sleepy, but because orthostatic intolerance prevents them from sitting comfortably for extended periods. Similarly, patients with MCAS might avoid situations that could trigger symptoms, skewing their scores.

Modified ESS for Autonomic Conditions includes:

Position-Specific Sleepiness Assessment:

- How likely are you to doze while lying flat (not just sitting)?
- What's your sleepiness level when properly supported with pillows?
- How does your sleepiness change with position changes?

Symptom-Adjusted Scenarios:

- How likely are you to fall asleep during activities you can actually tolerate?
- What's your sleepiness level on days when your other symptoms are well-controlled?
- How does symptom severity affect your daytime alertness?

This modification helps distinguish between true sleep debt and the complex fatigue patterns seen in autonomic dysfunction. Patients might be severely sleep-deprived but still unable to nap due to orthostatic intolerance or mast cell reactivity.

Pediatric Sleep Questionnaire Adaptations for Young Patients

Children with EDS, POTS, and MCAS face unique sleep challenges that standard pediatric assessments often miss. The Pediatric Sleep Questionnaire (PSQ) focuses primarily on sleep-disordered breathing and behavioral sleep problems, missing the joint instability and autonomic issues that plague young patients with these conditions (Chervin et al., 2000).

Enhanced PSQ for EDS/POTS/MCAS includes:

Developmental Considerations:

- Does your child complain of joints "coming apart" during sleep?
- Are there frequent position changes throughout the night?
- Does your child wake up with unexplained fears or anxiety?
- Are there predictable awakening times with physical symptoms?

Growth and Development Impacts:

- Has sleep disruption affected school performance?
- Are there concerns about growth or development?
- Does your child avoid sleepovers or overnight activities due to sleep problems?
- Are there family disruptions due to nighttime symptoms?

Children often can't articulate their sleep problems the way adults can, making observation-based assessment crucial. Parents need to become sleep detectives, tracking patterns and triggers that might not be obvious.

Home Assessment Protocols and Symptom Tracking

Professional sleep studies aren't always accessible or appropriate for patients with complex medical conditions. Home assessment protocols can provide valuable information and help patients become active participants in understanding their sleep patterns.

Daily Sleep Diary with Condition-Specific Tracking:

The standard sleep diary tracks bedtime, wake time, and sleep quality. Our enhanced version adds:

Pre-Sleep Assessment:

- Joint stability rating (1-10 scale)
- Autonomic symptom severity
- Mast cell symptom presence
- Position and support setup used

Awakening Documentation:

- Time and suspected cause of awakening
- Symptoms present upon awakening
- Ability to return to sleep
- Position changes needed

Morning Assessment:

- Joint status upon awakening
- Energy level and cognitive clarity
- Symptom flare presence
- Overall sleep satisfaction

This detailed tracking often reveals patterns that surprise both patients and providers. Many patients discover their sleep problems aren't random but follow predictable patterns related to their underlying conditions.

Differential Diagnosis Framework

Primary vs. Secondary Sleep Disorders

One of the biggest challenges in treating sleep problems in EDS, POTS, and MCAS patients is determining what's a primary sleep disorder versus what's secondary to the underlying condition. This distinction is crucial because treatment approaches differ dramatically.

Primary Sleep Disorders exist independently of the underlying condition and require specific sleep medicine interventions. These might include:

- Obstructive sleep apnea (which occurs at higher rates in EDS due to tissue laxity)
- Restless leg syndrome (beyond what's explained by MCAS)
- Periodic limb movement disorder
- Circadian rhythm disorders

Secondary Sleep Disruptions result directly from the underlying condition and require condition-specific management:

- POTS-related autonomic arousal preventing sleep onset
- EDS-related joint subluxations causing awakening
- MCAS-related histamine surges disrupting sleep architecture

The tricky part is that many patients have both primary and secondary sleep problems. A patient might have sleep apnea *and* joint instability *and* histamine surges. Each component needs appropriate treatment for optimal outcomes.

Red Flags Requiring Immediate Medical Attention

Certain sleep-related symptoms in this population require urgent evaluation because they may indicate life-threatening complications:

Cardiovascular Red Flags:

- New or worsening nighttime chest pain
- Severe palpitations with lightheadedness
- Episodes of suspected cardiac arrhythmia

- Signs of heart failure (orthopnea, paroxysmal nocturnal dyspnea)

Respiratory Red Flags:

- Witnessed apnea episodes (especially in EDS patients with tissue laxity)
- New or worsening breathing difficulties during sleep
- Choking or gasping episodes
- Cyanosis or color changes during sleep

Neurological Red Flags:

- New seizure-like activity during sleep
- Severe headaches upon awakening (possible intracranial pressure changes)
- Sudden onset of sleep paralysis or cataplexy
- Significant changes in cognitive function

Mast Cell Emergency Signs:

- Suspected anaphylaxis during sleep
- Severe breathing difficulties with flushing
- Loss of consciousness with mast cell symptoms
- Progressive worsening of nighttime reactions

These red flags require immediate medical evaluation, not gradual symptom management. The complex medical histories of these patients can make emergency assessment challenging, so clear documentation of baseline symptoms helps differentiate new problems from chronic issues.

Population-Specific Screening

POTS: Autonomic Arousal Patterns and Heart Rate Monitoring

POTS patients need specialized screening that captures the relationship between autonomic dysfunction and sleep disruption. Standard sleep questionnaires miss the nuanced ways that dysautonomia affects sleep architecture.

Heart Rate Variability Assessment: POTS patients often have abnormal heart rate patterns during sleep that don't show up on basic monitoring. Heart rate variability (HRV) measurement can reveal autonomic dysfunction that affects sleep quality even when heart rate appears normal.

Positional Sleep Assessment: The relationship between position and symptoms is crucial in POTS. Patients need screening that evaluates:

- Symptoms in different sleep positions
- Response to head-of-bed elevation
- Relationship between position changes and awakening
- Tolerance for supine positioning

Orthostatic Challenge During Sleep Assessment: Some patients develop orthostatic symptoms even from minor position changes during sleep. This requires evaluation of:

- Heart rate response to position changes during sleep
- Blood pressure changes with position
- Symptom development with elevation changes
- Recovery time from position-related symptoms

Sleep-Related Autonomic Symptoms: POTS-specific screening should assess:

- "Wired but tired" episodes
- Temperature regulation problems during sleep
- Digestive symptoms that disrupt sleep
- Cognitive symptoms upon awakening

EDS: Joint Position Assessment and Pain Documentation

EDS patients require screening that captures the complex relationship between joint instability and sleep disruption. This goes far beyond asking about pain levels.

Joint-Specific Sleep Assessment: Different joints present different challenges during sleep:

Shoulder Assessment:

- Frequency of shoulder subluxations during sleep
- Tolerance for side sleeping positions
- Need for supportive pillows or devices
- Morning shoulder pain or stiffness

Hip and Pelvis Assessment:

- SI joint pain that worsens with sleep position
- Hip instability in side-lying positions
- Need for pillow support between knees
- Morning hip stiffness or catching

Cervical Spine Assessment:

- Neck position tolerance during sleep
- Pillow requirements for neck support
- Morning headaches or neck pain
- Cervical instability symptoms

Temporomandibular Joint Assessment:

- Jaw clenching or grinding during sleep
- TMJ pain affecting sleep position
- Airway concerns related to jaw position
- Morning jaw pain or clicking

Sleep Position Tolerance: EDS patients need assessment of:

- Preferred and tolerated sleep positions

- Position changes needed during the night
- Use of supportive devices or pillows
- Relationship between position and symptom severity

MCAS: Histamine Surge Timing and Trigger Identification

MCAS patients require screening that captures the predictable patterns of mast cell activation that disrupt sleep. This includes both timing and trigger assessment.

Circadian Mast Cell Activity Assessment:

- Predictable awakening times (especially 2-4am)
- Symptoms present during nighttime awakening
- Seasonal variations in sleep disruption
- Relationship to menstrual cycles in women

Environmental Trigger Screening: MCAS patients need evaluation of bedroom environmental factors:

- Reaction to bedding materials
- Sensitivity to laundry detergents or fabric softeners
- Response to room temperature changes
- Reaction to air quality or humidity levels

Dietary Trigger Assessment:

- Relationship between evening meals and sleep disruption
- Response to histamine-containing foods
- Timing of last meal and sleep quality
- Alcohol or medication triggers

Stress and Emotional Trigger Evaluation:

- Relationship between stress levels and sleep quality
- Impact of emotional events on nighttime symptoms
- Response to relaxation techniques
- Effect of anticipatory anxiety on sleep

Documentation Strategies for Healthcare Providers

Healthcare providers need systematic approaches to document sleep problems in this population. Generic sleep assessments miss crucial information that guides treatment decisions.

Comprehensive Sleep History Should Include:

Timeline Development:

- When did sleep problems begin relative to other symptoms?
- How have sleep problems evolved over time?
- What interventions have been tried and their results?
- Relationship between sleep quality and overall symptom severity

Symptom Pattern Recognition:

- Are sleep problems episodic or continuous?
- What are the triggers for sleep disruption?
- How do sleep problems affect daytime functioning?
- What are the consequences of poor sleep on other symptoms?

Treatment Response Documentation:

- Which interventions have helped or worsened sleep?
- What medications or supplements have been tried?
- How do patients respond to positioning devices or environmental changes?
- What are the barriers to implementing effective interventions?

Functional Impact Assessment:

- How do sleep problems affect work or school performance?
- What is the impact on family relationships and social functioning?
- How does sleep quality affect overall quality of life?

- What adaptations has the patient made to cope with sleep problems?

The goal isn't just to document problems but to identify patterns that guide treatment decisions. Effective screening in this population requires understanding the complex interactions between multiple pathophysiological processes and their impact on sleep architecture.

Straight Talk on Assessment Reality

The biggest problem with sleep assessment in EDS, POTS, and MCAS isn't that we don't have tools — it's that we're not using the right tools systematically. Most healthcare providers rely on quick questions that miss the complexity of sleep problems in these conditions.

Patients often need to become their own sleep detectives, tracking patterns and triggers that their healthcare providers might miss. This isn't ideal, but it's the current reality. The detailed assessment tools described here can help patients advocate for appropriate care and guide their own management strategies.

Key Assessment Strategies:

- Use condition-specific modifications of standard sleep questionnaires to capture relevant symptoms
- Implement detailed home tracking to identify patterns that might not be apparent during brief medical visits
- Differentiate between primary sleep disorders requiring sleep medicine interventions and secondary sleep disruptions needing condition-specific management
- Recognize red flag symptoms that require immediate medical evaluation
- Document functional impact and treatment responses to guide ongoing management decisions

Chapter 3: The Science of Sleep Disruption in Connective Tissue and Autonomic Disorders

The sleep problems plaguing patients with EDS, POTS, and MCAS aren't mysterious or psychological — they're the predictable result of well-understood pathophysiological mechanisms. Yet the medical community continues to treat these sleep disruptions as minor inconveniences rather than serious manifestations of underlying disease processes. This disconnect between scientific knowledge and clinical practice is both frustrating and dangerous.

Understanding the mechanisms behind sleep disruption in these conditions isn't just academic exercise — it's the foundation for effective treatment. When you understand *why* your shoulder subluxates at 3am or *why* you wake up with a racing heart at predictable times, you can develop targeted interventions instead of hoping that generic sleep advice will somehow work.

Pathophysiology Deep Dive

Proprioceptive Dysfunction and Sleep Position Challenges

Proprioception — your body's ability to sense joint position and movement — is fundamentally impaired in patients with EDS and related connective tissue disorders. This isn't just about being "flexible" or "double-jointed." It's about having defective sensory feedback systems that normally prevent injury during movement and position changes (Rombaut et al., 2010).

During waking hours, patients with EDS compensate for poor proprioception through visual feedback, conscious attention to joint position, and muscle guarding. But during sleep, these compensatory mechanisms shut down, leaving joints vulnerable to subluxation and dislocation with even minor position changes.

The problem starts with defective collagen affecting the mechanoreceptors in joint capsules, ligaments, and tendons. These sensors normally provide continuous feedback about joint position and load. When this feedback system is impaired, the brain doesn't receive accurate information about joint stress or position, leading to movements that exceed safe ranges of motion.

The Sleep-Specific Vulnerability: During REM sleep, voluntary muscle tone decreases dramatically, leaving joints dependent on passive stability from ligaments and joint capsules. In EDS patients, these structures are inherently weak and overstretched. The combination of reduced muscle tone and defective passive restraints creates a perfect storm for nighttime subluxations.

Research has documented that patients with joint hypermobility show significantly impaired position sense even when awake and alert (Rombaut et al., 2010). During sleep, this impairment becomes even more pronounced, leading to position changes that would trigger immediate protective responses in people with normal proprioception.

Specific Joint Vulnerabilities During Sleep:

Shoulder Complex: The glenohumeral joint depends heavily on muscular stability, which decreases during sleep. Side sleeping puts the dependent shoulder at risk for anterior subluxation, while the upper shoulder can subluxate posteriorly from pillow pressure or arm positioning.

Cervical Spine: Neck position during sleep affects multiple structures — the atlantooccipital joint, suboccipital muscles, and the cervical facet joints. Poor pillow support can lead to hyperextension, hyperflexion, or rotation that exceeds safe ranges.

Hip and Pelvis: The sacroiliac joints are particularly vulnerable in side-lying positions without proper support. Hip external rotation combined with adduction can strain the joint capsule and surrounding ligaments.

Temporomandibular Joint: Jaw position during sleep affects not only TMJ stability but also airway patency. Patients with EDS often have increased TMJ mobility that predisposes to subluxation during sleep.

Autonomic Nervous System Dysregulation Mechanisms

The autonomic dysfunction in POTS creates a cascade of sleep-disrupting mechanisms that operate at multiple levels. This isn't simple "anxiety" or "stress" — it's documented physiological dysfunction affecting the fundamental processes that regulate sleep-wake cycles.

Sympathetic Hyperactivity and Sleep Onset: POTS patients often demonstrate elevated sympathetic activity even at rest, which directly interferes with the normal transition to sleep. The parasympathetic dominance required for sleep onset is compromised by persistent sympathetic arousal (Bagai et al., 2011).

Heart rate variability studies in POTS patients show reduced parasympathetic activity and increased sympathetic predominance, particularly during evening hours when the nervous system should be shifting toward restorative parasympathetic dominance. This creates the "wired but tired" phenomenon — physical exhaustion combined with physiological arousal that prevents sleep.

Thermoregulatory Dysfunction: Normal sleep involves a decrease in core body temperature, mediated by autonomic control of peripheral vasodilation. POTS patients often have impaired thermoregulation due to dysfunction of the sympathetic nerves controlling blood vessel diameter and sweat production.

The result is difficulty achieving the temperature drop necessary for sleep onset, unpredictable night sweats that disrupt sleep, and sensitivity to ambient temperature changes that would barely affect people with normal autonomic function. Some patients report feeling simultaneously hot and cold, or experiencing temperature fluctuations that seem unrelated to environmental conditions.

Cardiovascular Arousal Patterns: The cardiovascular manifestations of POTS don't stop during sleep. Heart rate increases with position changes, blood pressure fluctuations occur with minor stimuli, and cardiac output changes unpredictably. These cardiovascular changes often wake patients or prevent deep sleep.

Nocturnal tachycardia is particularly problematic because it can trigger anxiety responses that further activate the sympathetic nervous system, creating a cycle of arousal that can last for hours. Some patients develop conditioned anxiety about sleep itself, further complicating the autonomic dysfunction.

Gastrointestinal Autonomic Dysfunction: The autonomic nervous system controls digestive function, and POTS patients frequently experience gastroparesis, intestinal dysmotility, and other GI problems that disrupt sleep. Nocturnal nausea, abdominal pain, and unpredictable bowel function can cause awakening and prevent return to sleep.

The relationship between autonomic dysfunction and sleep is bidirectional — poor sleep worsens autonomic function, while autonomic dysfunction prevents good sleep. Breaking this cycle requires targeted interventions that address the underlying physiological dysfunction, not just symptom management.

Mast Cell Circadian Rhythm Disruption

Mast cells have their own circadian rhythm, with peak degranulation occurring in the early morning hours when cortisol levels are rising. This isn't coincidental — it reflects evolutionary programming that prepared our ancestors for the stress of starting a new day. But in patients with MCAS, this normal circadian pattern becomes pathological.

The 2-4am Histamine Surge Phenomenon: Research has documented that plasma histamine levels show circadian variation in healthy individuals, with peak levels occurring between 2-4am

(Nakamura et al., 2017). In patients with MCAS, this normal pattern is amplified to pathological levels, creating predictable sleep disruption.

The timing isn't random — it corresponds to the circadian rise in cortisol and other stress hormones. In healthy individuals, this provides gentle arousal to prepare for waking. In MCAS patients, it triggers full mast cell degranulation with symptoms severe enough to cause complete awakening.

Molecular Mechanisms of Circadian Mast Cell Activity: Mast cells contain circadian clock genes (CLOCK, PER2, CRY1) that regulate their activation patterns. These genes control the expression of enzymes involved in histamine synthesis and the sensitivity of degranulation pathways (Nakamura et al., 2017).

The organic cation transporter 3 (OCT3), which helps clear histamine from tissues, also shows circadian variation. During early morning hours, OCT3 activity is at its lowest, meaning histamine persists longer in tissues and creates more potent symptoms.

Triggers for Nocturnal Mast Cell Activation: Several factors can trigger or amplify the normal circadian pattern of mast cell activity:

Temperature Changes: The normal circadian drop in body temperature can trigger mast cell degranulation in sensitive individuals. This explains why some patients react to air conditioning, fan use, or simply cooling off during sleep.

Hormonal Fluctuations: Cortisol, growth hormone, and other hormones that fluctuate during sleep can trigger mast cell activation. The timing of these fluctuations often coincides with patient reports of predictable awakening times.

Stress Response: Even during sleep, the nervous system responds to internal and external stressors. In MCAS patients, normal stress responses can trigger mast cell degranulation that disrupts sleep.

Food and Chemical Exposures: Delayed reactions to foods, medications, or environmental chemicals can manifest during sleep hours, particularly during the vulnerable early morning period when mast cell activity peaks.

The Inflammatory Sleep Disruption Cycle

All three conditions — EDS, POTS, and MCAS — involve inflammatory processes that both disrupt sleep and are worsened by poor sleep. This creates a vicious cycle where sleep problems worsen inflammation, which further disrupts sleep.

Sleep Deprivation and Inflammatory Markers: Chronic sleep disruption increases inflammatory cytokines (IL-6, TNF-alpha, CRP) and decreases anti-inflammatory mediators. This systemic inflammation worsens joint pain in EDS, autonomic dysfunction in POTS, and mast cell reactivity in MCAS.

Pain-Sleep Interaction: Joint pain and instability in EDS create sleep disruption, but sleep deprivation also lowers pain thresholds and increases pain sensitivity. This bidirectional relationship means that addressing either pain or sleep problems alone is often insufficient — both must be targeted simultaneously.

Autonomic-Inflammatory Connections: The autonomic nervous system regulates inflammatory responses through the cholinergic anti-inflammatory pathway. Dysfunction of this system in POTS patients can lead to increased systemic inflammation that further disrupts sleep and worsens symptoms.

Medical Evidence vs. Patient Experience

What Studies Definitively Prove

The research base supporting the mechanisms described above is solid, though not complete. We have definitive evidence for several key points:

Documented Sleep Architecture Changes: Polysomnographic studies in POTS patients show measurable changes in sleep architecture — increased sleep latency, reduced REM sleep, increased sleep fragmentation, and abnormal autonomic activity during sleep (Bagai et al., 2011).

Circadian Mast Cell Activity: Multiple studies have documented circadian variation in mast cell mediator levels and the expression of circadian clock genes in mast cells (Nakamura et al., 2017). The 2-4am peak in histamine activity is well-established.

Proprioceptive Deficits in EDS: Research has consistently demonstrated impaired position sense and joint position awareness in patients with joint hypermobility syndromes (Rombaut et al., 2010). These deficits affect both static position sense and dynamic movement awareness.

Sleep-Inflammation Relationships: The bidirectional relationship between sleep quality and inflammatory markers is well-documented in multiple populations, including patients with chronic pain and autoimmune conditions.

Areas of Ongoing Medical Controversy

Despite solid evidence for basic mechanisms, several areas remain controversial or understudied:

The EDS-POTS-MCAS Connection: While clinical observation suggests these conditions frequently occur together, the mechanistic relationships aren't fully understood. Some researchers question whether they represent distinct conditions or different manifestations of a shared underlying pathophysiology.

Mast Cell Activation Syndrome Validity: Some medical professionals question the validity of MCAS as a distinct diagnosis, arguing that mast cell activation is a normal response to various stimuli rather than a pathological condition. This controversy affects diagnosis and treatment access.

Sleep Intervention Efficacy: While we understand the mechanisms of sleep disruption, we have limited research on the efficacy of specific interventions. Most treatment recommendations are based on clinical experience rather than randomized controlled trials.

Genetic vs. Acquired Factors: The relative contributions of genetic predisposition versus acquired factors (infections, trauma, stress) in developing these conditions remain unclear. This affects both understanding of disease mechanisms and treatment approaches.

Patient-Reported Patterns Awaiting Research Validation

Patients consistently report patterns and experiences that haven't been formally studied but deserve research attention:

Predictable Symptom Timing: Patients report remarkably consistent timing of symptoms — the 2-4am awakening pattern in MCAS, the evening worsening of POTS symptoms, the morning stiffness patterns in EDS. These observations suggest circadian factors that haven't been fully investigated.

Environmental Sensitivity Patterns: Patients report specific environmental triggers that affect sleep — weather changes, barometric pressure, seasonal variations. These reports suggest mechanisms that aren't well understood by conventional medicine.

Medication Response Patterns: Patients often report unusual responses to medications — paradoxical reactions to sedatives, unexpected benefits from medications not typically used for sleep, timing-dependent effects. These patterns suggest pharmacokinetic or pharmacodynamic differences that haven't been studied.

Multi-Generational Patterns: Many patients report family histories of similar sleep problems, suggesting genetic factors that haven't been systematically investigated.

Navigating Medical Skepticism While Seeking Care

The gap between patient experience and medical recognition creates challenges for obtaining appropriate care. Many patients face skepticism from healthcare providers who aren't familiar with these conditions or who question the validity of patient reports.

Strategies for Effective Medical Communication:

Document Patterns: Keep detailed records of symptoms, timing, triggers, and responses to interventions. Objective documentation is more persuasive than subjective reports.

Bring Research: Print relevant studies that support your reported experiences. Many providers aren't familiar with the literature on these conditions.

Request Specific Testing: Ask for heart rate variability studies, sleep studies with autonomic monitoring, or mast cell mediator testing. Objective test results are harder to dismiss than subjective reports.

Seek Specialist Care: Find providers who specialize in these conditions and understand their complexity. General practitioners often lack the expertise to manage these conditions effectively.

Join Patient Communities: Connect with other patients who can share successful strategies for obtaining care and managing symptoms.

The science supporting the sleep disruption mechanisms in EDS, POTS, and MCAS is solid enough to guide treatment decisions, even if all the details aren't worked out. Patients can't afford to wait for perfect research when effective interventions are available based on current understanding.

The Research We Still Need

While our understanding of sleep disruption mechanisms has advanced significantly, important gaps remain:

Intervention Studies: We need randomized controlled trials of specific interventions for sleep problems in these populations. Most current recommendations are based on case series or clinical experience.

Biomarker Studies: Research into objective biomarkers that predict sleep problems or treatment response could help guide personalized interventions.

Long-term Outcome Studies: We need data on the long-term effects of sleep interventions on overall disease progression and quality of life.

Mechanistic Studies: Research into the specific pathways connecting tissue abnormalities, autonomic dysfunction, and mast cell activation could lead to more targeted treatments.

Time for Intellectual Honesty

The mechanisms underlying sleep disruption in EDS, POTS, and MCAS are well enough understood to guide effective interventions. The problem isn't lack of knowledge — it's lack of application of existing knowledge to clinical practice.

Patients experiencing these sleep problems aren't suffering from poor sleep hygiene or psychological issues — they're dealing with predictable physiological dysfunction that requires targeted interventions. The sooner we acknowledge this reality and act accordingly, the sooner we can help people get the restorative sleep they desperately need.

The next chapter will address the emergency protocols needed when sleep disruption becomes dangerous, because understanding mechanisms is meaningless if we're not prepared to handle the serious complications that can arise.

Critical Understanding Points:

- Sleep problems in EDS, POTS, and MCAS result from well-documented physiological mechanisms, not psychological factors
- Proprioceptive dysfunction in EDS creates predictable joint instability during sleep that can be prevented with proper positioning
- Autonomic dysfunction in POTS causes measurable sleep architecture changes that require targeted interventions
- Mast cell circadian rhythms create predictable 2-4am symptom patterns that can be managed with appropriate protocols
- The bidirectional relationship between sleep and inflammation means both must be addressed simultaneously for optimal outcomes

Chapter 4: Nocturnal Emergency Response Systems

The middle of the night isn't exactly prime time for medical emergencies, but tell that to your mast cells at 3am or your shoulder that's just decided to subluxate while you're dead asleep. These conditions don't follow convenient business hours, and the emergency room staff probably won't appreciate your detailed explanation of why your symptoms aren't "just anxiety" at two in the morning. So you need to be prepared — really prepared — because when things go wrong during sleep, they can go very wrong, very fast.

Most people think emergency preparedness means having a first aid kit somewhere in the house (probably expired) and maybe knowing how to call 911. That's cute, but it won't cut it for patients with EDS, POTS, and MCAS. You need protocols, not panic. You need systems, not scrambling. And you need to know exactly what constitutes a real emergency versus what you can handle at home, because the difference can mean everything.

Life-Threatening Events Management

Nocturnal Anaphylaxis Emergency Protocol

Anaphylaxis during sleep is the nightmare scenario that every MCAS patient fears — and for good reason. You're unconscious, your protective reflexes are dampened, and your mast cells can dump their entire contents without warning. The American Academy of Family Physicians reports that anaphylaxis can progress from initial symptoms to cardiovascular collapse in as little as 10-15 minutes (Lieberman et al., 2015). During sleep, you might miss those early warning signs entirely.

The first problem with nocturnal anaphylaxis is recognition. You might wake up already in the middle of a severe reaction, confused and disoriented from sleep, trying to figure out what's happening while your blood pressure is dropping and your airways are constricting. This isn't the time for careful differential diagnosis.

Step-by-Step Nocturnal Anaphylaxis Protocol:

1. **Immediate Recognition Signs**
   - Sudden awakening with sense of impending doom
   - Difficulty breathing or throat tightness
   - Rapid onset of widespread hives or flushing
   - Dizziness, lightheadedness, or feeling faint
   - Nausea, vomiting, or severe abdominal cramping
   - Rapid heart rate or palpitations
2. **First Response Actions (Within 60 seconds)**
   - Sit up or elevate head of bed immediately
   - Administer epinephrine auto-injector without hesitation
   - Call 911 or have your partner call immediately
   - Take fast-acting antihistamines if you can swallow safely
   - Start continuous monitoring of your condition
3. **Secondary Support Measures**
   - Remove any potential triggers from immediate environment
   - Prepare for second epinephrine dose (may be needed in 10-15 minutes)
   - Document time of onset and interventions taken
   - Prepare medication list and medical history for emergency responders
   - Stay calm but stay vigilant — anaphylaxis can be biphasic

The key point here is that you treat first and ask questions later. If you wake up with signs that could be anaphylaxis, you use your epinephrine immediately. You don't wait to see if it gets worse. You don't wonder if it's really that serious. You don't debate whether you're overreacting. Epinephrine won't hurt you if you don't need it, but waiting when you do need it can kill you.

Biphasic Anaphylaxis Awareness: Here's what makes nocturnal anaphylaxis particularly dangerous — up to 20% of anaphylactic reactions are biphasic, meaning symptoms improve initially but then return 4-12 hours later, sometimes more severely (Ellis & Day, 2003). If you have an anaphylactic reaction during the night, you're not out of the woods just because the epinephrine worked. You need emergency medical evaluation and extended monitoring.

POTS Crisis Management During Sleep

POTS crises during sleep present differently than daytime episodes but can be equally dangerous. The Cleveland Clinic documents that severe POTS episodes can involve heart rates exceeding 120 beats per minute with position changes, blood pressure instability, and risk of syncope (Sheldon et al., 2015). During sleep, these episodes often manifest as sudden awakening with severe tachycardia, chest discomfort, and overwhelming anxiety.

Recognizing Nocturnal POTS Crisis:

- Sudden awakening with heart racing (often >120 bpm)
- Chest pain or pressure sensation
- Severe dizziness or feeling like you might faint
- Overwhelming sense of panic or impending doom
- Nausea or gastrointestinal distress
- Profuse sweating or feeling overheated
- Trembling or shaking

Immediate Management Protocol:

1. **Position Management**
   - Stay lying down initially — don't sit up quickly
   - Elevate legs above heart level if possible
   - Avoid sudden position changes
   - Keep head elevated to prevent blood pooling
2. **Rapid Intervention**
   - Drink fluids immediately (keep water at bedside)
   - Take salt tablets or drink electrolyte solution

- o Use compression garments if available nearby
- o Begin slow, controlled breathing techniques
3. **Monitoring and Decision Making**
    - o Check heart rate and blood pressure if possible
    - o Monitor for chest pain or severe symptoms
    - o Assess ability to speak and think clearly
    - o Determine if symptoms are improving with interventions

When to Call 911 for POTS Crisis:

- Heart rate remains >150 bpm after 10 minutes of intervention
- Chest pain is severe or worsening
- You lose consciousness or nearly lose consciousness
- Symptoms don't improve with standard interventions
- You develop new symptoms like severe shortness of breath

The tricky part about POTS crises is that they can feel like heart attacks or other cardiac emergencies. Don't try to be a hero and tough it out if you're genuinely concerned about cardiac symptoms. Emergency rooms see POTS patients regularly, and while the experience might be frustrating, it's better than missing a real cardiac event.

Joint Dislocation and Subluxation Safe Reduction

Joint subluxations during sleep are remarkably common in EDS patients, but the approach to managing them at night requires careful consideration. The Ehlers-Danlos Society emphasizes that while many patients become skilled at reducing their own subluxations, nighttime reductions carry additional risks due to decreased awareness and potential for further injury (Malfait et al., 2017).

Common Nocturnal Subluxation Sites:

- Shoulders (most frequent, particularly anterior subluxation)
- Hips and SI joints
- Ribs (often multiple ribs at once)

- Cervical spine
- Temporomandibular joints

Safe Self-Reduction Principles:

1. **Assessment Before Action**
   - Are you fully awake and alert?
   - Is the subluxation in a location you've successfully reduced before?
   - Do you have adequate support and positioning available?
   - Are there any new or unusual symptoms?
2. **Gentle Reduction Techniques**
   - Use minimal force — if it doesn't reduce easily, stop
   - Support the joint during and after reduction
   - Move slowly and deliberately
   - Listen to your body — pain is a warning signal
3. **Post-Reduction Care**
   - Stabilize the joint with pillows or supports
   - Ice if there's significant pain or swelling
   - Monitor for return of stability
   - Document the episode for pattern recognition

When NOT to Attempt Self-Reduction:

- Complete dislocation rather than subluxation
- Numbness or tingling in the extremity
- Loss of circulation (pale, blue, or cold limb)
- Severe pain that doesn't improve with position changes
- Multiple joints affected simultaneously
- Any spinal involvement with neurological symptoms

Emergency Situations Requiring Immediate Medical Care:

- Shoulder dislocation with arm numbness
- Hip dislocation that doesn't reduce easily
- Cervical spine involvement with any neurological symptoms
- Rib dislocations affecting breathing

- Any subluxation with loss of circulation

The reality is that most experienced EDS patients become quite skilled at managing their routine subluxations. But nighttime episodes can be tricky because you're not fully alert, you might not have optimal positioning, and you could miss warning signs of more serious injury. When in doubt, err on the side of caution and seek medical evaluation.

Decision Tree for Emergency vs. Home Management

The hardest part of nocturnal emergencies is often deciding what requires emergency care versus what you can manage at home. Here's a framework for making these decisions quickly and accurately:

Immediate 911 Situations (No Discussion Needed):

- Anaphylaxis signs (breathing difficulty, widespread reaction, circulation problems)
- Loss of consciousness or near-loss of consciousness
- Severe chest pain with sweating and nausea
- Complete inability to breathe or severe breathing distress
- Severe injury with deformity or loss of function
- Any situation where you feel you might die or be permanently harmed

Emergency Room Within 1-2 Hours:

- Suspected complete joint dislocation that won't reduce
- Heart rate >150 bpm that doesn't respond to usual interventions
- Severe allergic reaction that partially responds to antihistamines but doesn't fully resolve
- Joint subluxation with numbness, tingling, or circulation changes
- Severe pain that's different from your usual patterns

Urgent Care or Doctor Visit Within 24 Hours:

- Joint subluxations that reduce but keep recurring

- POTS symptoms that are more severe than usual but respond to interventions
- Allergic reactions that resolve with antihistamines but concern you
- Sleep disruptions that represent a significant change in your pattern
- Any symptoms that worry you but aren't immediately life-threatening

Home Management Appropriate:

- Routine subluxations that reduce easily and stay reduced
- Mild to moderate POTS symptoms that respond to your usual interventions
- Histamine reactions that respond well to antihistamines
- Sleep disruptions that follow your usual patterns
- Symptoms that are consistent with your baseline condition

Emergency Medication Administration

Bedside Emergency Kit Setup and Maintenance

Every patient with these conditions needs a bedside emergency kit — not just medications thrown in a drawer, but a properly organized, easily accessible system that works even when you're half-awake and panicked. Your emergency kit is useless if you can't find what you need in the dark or if everything is expired.

Essential Bedside Emergency Kit Contents:

Anaphylaxis Response:

- Two epinephrine auto-injectors (always have backup)
- Fast-acting liquid antihistamine (Benadryl liquid works faster than tablets)
- Oral corticosteroids (prednisone or methylprednisolone)
- Albuterol inhaler for breathing symptoms
- Medical alert information and emergency contacts

POTS Crisis Management:

- Oral electrolyte supplements or salt tablets
- Sports drink or electrolyte powder for quick mixing
- Blood pressure cuff and pulse oximeter if you have them
- Emergency phone numbers for your cardiologist or POTS specialist
- Compression stockings or garments

EDS Emergency Supplies:

- Instant ice packs for acute injuries
- Elastic bandages for joint support
- Pain medications (both prescription and over-the-counter)
- Thermometer for monitoring fever with injuries
- Emergency phone numbers for orthopedic contacts

Organization and Maintenance:

- Use a clear plastic container that's easy to grab
- Label everything clearly with expiration dates
- Check expiration dates monthly and replace as needed
- Keep emergency kit within arm's reach of your bed
- Make sure your partner knows where everything is located

Epinephrine Auto-Injector Protocols

The new nasal spray epinephrine formulations have changed the game for anaphylaxis treatment, but many patients and even healthcare providers aren't familiar with proper usage protocols. The key advantage of nasal epinephrine is that it doesn't require injection, making it easier to use during severe reactions when fine motor skills might be impaired.

Traditional Auto-Injector Protocol:

1. Remove from case immediately when needed
2. Pull off blue safety cap

3. Place orange tip against outer thigh
4. Push firmly until you hear the click
5. Hold for 10 seconds
6. Massage injection site for 10 seconds
7. Call 911 immediately after administration

Nasal Spray Epinephrine Protocol:

1. Remove cap and insert device in nostril
2. Press plunger firmly to deliver full dose
3. Repeat in other nostril if available
4. Onset of action may be slightly slower than injection
5. Call 911 immediately after administration

Critical Timing Considerations: The American Academy of Family Physicians emphasizes that epinephrine should be administered at the first sign of anaphylaxis, not as a last resort (Lieberman et al., 2015). Many patients wait too long, hoping symptoms will improve on their own. This delay can be fatal.

Common Mistakes to Avoid:

- Waiting to see if antihistamines work first
- Using expired auto-injectors (replace annually)
- Injecting through thick clothing (though possible, direct skin contact is better)
- Forgetting to call 911 after using epinephrine
- Not having a second dose available for biphasic reactions

Fast-Acting Antihistamine Administration

The speed of antihistamine absorption can make the difference between a manageable reaction and a medical emergency. Liquid formulations work faster than tablets, sublingual tablets work faster than swallowed pills, and IV antihistamines work fastest of all (though that's obviously not an option for home use).

Optimal Antihistamine Protocol for Nocturnal Reactions:

1. **First-line response:** Liquid diphenhydramine (Benadryl) 25-50mg
2. **Secondary H2 blocker:** Famotidine (Pepcid) 20mg if you can swallow
3. **Mast cell stabilizer:** Quercetin or cromolyn if part of your regimen
4. **Monitor response:** Symptoms should begin improving within 15-30 minutes

Absorption Enhancement Strategies:

- Take on empty stomach if possible (faster absorption)
- Use liquid formulations for severe reactions
- Consider sublingual tablets for patients with gastroparesis
- Dissolve regular tablets in small amount of water if necessary

Partner and Caregiver Training Requirements

Your emergency protocols are only as good as the people around you who might need to implement them. If you live with someone, they need to know what to do — not just theoretically, but practically. They need to know where everything is, how to use it, and when to call for help.

Essential Partner Training Topics:

Recognition Training:

- What does anaphylaxis look like in you specifically?
- How do your POTS crises typically present?
- What are your usual vs. emergency-level joint problems?
- When should they intervene vs. let you handle it?

Medication Administration:

- How to use epinephrine auto-injectors
- Proper antihistamine dosing and timing
- When to give additional medications

- How to document what was given and when

Emergency Response:

- When to call 911 vs. other emergency numbers
- What information to give emergency responders
- How to advocate for appropriate care in emergency settings
- How to locate and provide your medical information

Practical Scenarios:

- Practice using expired auto-injectors on oranges
- Role-play different emergency scenarios
- Review emergency contacts and medication lists regularly
- Practice finding emergency supplies in the dark

Medical Alert Systems and Monitoring

Device Selection Criteria for Each Condition

Medical alert systems for patients with complex conditions need to go beyond the basic "I've fallen and can't get up" model. You need systems that can communicate the complexity of your conditions and get appropriate help quickly. MedicAlert Foundation reports that patients with multiple medical conditions have significantly better emergency outcomes when they have properly configured medical alert systems (MedicAlert Foundation, 2018).

POTS-Specific Alert System Needs:

- Heart rate monitoring capabilities
- Fall detection (orthostatic episodes can cause falls)
- GPS location services (for episodes away from home)
- Direct connection to emergency services with medical history access
- Integration with cardiac monitoring if you use wearable devices

MCAS-Specific Alert System Features:

- Rapid response capability (anaphylaxis develops quickly)
- Medication administration tracking
- Allergy and trigger information readily available
- Connection to allergist or immunologist if available
- Environmental trigger tracking integration

EDS-Specific Alert Considerations:

- Joint injury documentation capabilities
- Physical therapy or orthopedic specialist contacts
- Pain level tracking and reporting
- Mobility assistance coordination
- Integration with imaging or specialist appointments

Multi-Condition Integration: The best systems for patients with all three conditions combine monitoring capabilities with rapid emergency response and detailed medical information access. Look for systems that:

- Allow detailed medical history input
- Provide 24/7 monitoring with trained medical personnel
- Integrate with your existing healthcare team
- Offer family notification options
- Include medication and allergy information

Integration with Healthcare Teams

Your emergency preparedness isn't just about what you do at home — it's about how well your emergency protocols integrate with your broader healthcare team. This means making sure your specialists know about your emergency experiences and that emergency responders can access your medical information quickly.

Healthcare Team Integration Strategies:

Primary Care Coordination:

- Provide your primary care doctor with copies of your emergency protocols
- Update emergency contact information regularly
- Share documentation of emergency episodes for pattern recognition
- Coordinate medication refills for emergency supplies

Specialist Communication:

- Make sure your POTS cardiologist knows about cardiac emergency episodes
- Keep your allergist informed about anaphylaxis episodes and triggers
- Share joint emergency episodes with orthopedic specialists or rheumatologists
- Coordinate emergency protocols with all your specialists

Emergency Medical Services:

- Consider registering with local EMS if your area offers this service
- Provide emergency contact information to local fire and police departments
- Keep updated medication and allergy lists easily accessible
- Consider medical alert jewelry or wallet cards with essential information

Cost-Effectiveness Analysis and Insurance Coverage

Medical alert systems and emergency preparedness supplies represent a significant investment, but the cost of not being prepared can be much higher. Emergency room visits, ambulance transport, and hospital admissions are expensive — and that's before you consider the cost of complications from delayed treatment.

Cost Comparison Analysis:

- Basic medical alert system: $30-60 per month

- Advanced monitoring system: $60-150 per month
- Emergency room visit: $1,500-5,000 per visit
- Ambulance transport: $500-2,000 per trip
- Hospital admission: $2,000-10,000 per day

Insurance Coverage Options:

- Some insurance plans cover medical alert systems for high-risk patients
- Medicare covers certain types of medical alert devices
- Flexible spending accounts can often be used for emergency preparedness supplies
- Some employers offer medical alert system benefits
- Disability insurance may cover monitoring systems in some cases

Return on Investment Calculations: If your medical alert system prevents just one unnecessary emergency room visit per year, it pays for itself. If it helps you get appropriate treatment faster during a real emergency, it could save your life. The cost-effectiveness analysis strongly favors investment in proper emergency preparedness for patients with these conditions.

The Reality of Emergency Preparedness

The truth about emergency preparedness for EDS, POTS, and MCAS patients is that you can't rely on the medical system to understand your conditions or respond appropriately to your crises. You need to be your own emergency medical technician, at least initially. This means having the right supplies, knowing how to use them, and having protocols that work even when you're scared, confused, or half-asleep.

Emergency preparedness isn't paranoia — it's practical planning for documented risks. The research shows that patients with these conditions have higher rates of emergency situations, more complex presentations, and greater risk of being misunderstood or mismanaged in emergency settings. Being prepared isn't just smart; it's essential for your safety and well-being.

The next chapter will focus specifically on the 2-4am crisis phenomenon that affects so many MCAS patients, because understanding and managing these predictable episodes can prevent many emergency situations entirely.

Emergency Preparedness Essentials:

- Develop condition-specific emergency protocols that account for the unique risks of EDS, POTS, and MCAS
- Maintain properly stocked and organized bedside emergency kits with medications and supplies that are easily accessible even in the dark
- Train partners and caregivers on recognition and response protocols specific to your conditions
- Choose medical alert systems that can communicate the complexity of your medical conditions to emergency responders
- Integrate emergency preparedness with your broader healthcare team to ensure continuity of care
- Calculate the cost-effectiveness of emergency preparedness — it pays for itself by preventing complications and unnecessary emergency visits

Chapter 5: The 2-4am Crisis Protocol

There's something uniquely cruel about mast cells having their own internal alarm clock set for the worst possible time. Just as you've finally achieved some semblance of deep sleep, your body decides it's the perfect moment to dump a pharmacy's worth of inflammatory mediators into your system. The 2-4am histamine surge isn't some mystical phenomenon — it's a well-documented, predictable pattern that affects nearly every MCAS patient, yet most healthcare providers have never heard of it.

This isn't random bad luck or poor sleep hygiene. Your mast cells are following their circadian programming, releasing mediators at times that would have made sense for our prehistoric ancestors but create misery for modern patients trying to get restorative sleep. The good news is that predictable problems have predictable solutions — if you understand the mechanisms and implement targeted interventions.

Understanding Nocturnal Histamine Surges

Circadian Mast Cell Activation Patterns

Mast cells don't just randomly decide to cause trouble in the middle of the night. They're following ancient biological programming controlled by circadian clock genes that regulate when cells are most active and reactive. Research published in Scientific Reports demonstrates that mast cells contain intrinsic circadian clocks that control both spontaneous degranulation and sensitivity to triggers (Nakamura et al., 2017).

The timing isn't coincidental — it corresponds to the natural circadian rise in cortisol and other stress hormones that occurs in the early morning hours. In healthy individuals, this gradual hormonal increase helps prepare the body for waking and the day's activities. But in MCAS patients, these same hormonal changes trigger massive mast cell degranulation that disrupts sleep and creates hours of misery.

The Molecular Clock Mechanism: Mast cells express the core circadian clock genes CLOCK, BMAL1, PER1, PER2, and CRY1/CRY2. These genes create oscillating patterns of protein expression that control cellular activity over 24-hour cycles. During the early morning hours (typically 2-4am), these clock genes drive increased expression of degranulation pathways and decreased expression of stabilizing factors.

Histamine Release Patterns: Studies show that plasma histamine levels in healthy individuals peak between 2-4am, but the levels are relatively modest and don't typically cause symptoms (Nakamura et al., 2017). In MCAS patients, this normal pattern is amplified dramatically, creating histamine surges that can be 10-20 times higher than baseline levels.

Organic Cation Transporter 3 (OCT3) Rhythms: The story gets more complicated when you consider histamine clearance. OCT3 is the main transporter responsible for removing histamine from tissues, and it also shows circadian variation. During the early morning hours, OCT3 activity is at its lowest, meaning histamine persists longer in tissues even after mast cells stop releasing it actively.

This creates a perfect storm — peak histamine release combined with minimal histamine clearance. The result is sustained high tissue histamine levels that can persist for hours, explaining why patients often can't get back to sleep after a 2-4am episode.

Evidence-Based Timing of Interventions

The predictable timing of nocturnal histamine surges allows for strategic intervention timing that can prevent or minimize episodes. The key is understanding that you need to have medications on board *before* the surge begins, not after you're already symptomatic.

Pre-emptive Medication Timing: Research suggests that H1 and H2 antihistamines reach peak effectiveness 1-2 hours after administration. This means taking your evening antihistamines at 11pm-midnight gives you maximum protection during the vulnerable 2-4am window.

Waiting until you're already symptomatic means you're trying to treat a problem that's already fully developed.

Mast Cell Stabilizer Timing: Medications like quercetin, cromolyn sodium, or ketotifen work by preventing mast cell degranulation rather than blocking histamine after it's released. These need to be on board well before the surge occurs — ideally 2-4 hours before your typical episode time. For most patients, this means taking mast cell stabilizers around 10pm-11pm.

Hormonal Consideration: The cortisol rise that triggers mast cell activation begins around midnight and peaks around 2-4am. Some patients benefit from very low-dose melatonin (0.5-1mg) taken around 10pm to help modulate this cortisol response. Higher doses of melatonin can actually worsen symptoms in some MCAS patients, so less is often more.

Environmental Trigger Management

The 2-4am time period represents peak vulnerability to environmental triggers that might not cause problems during other times of day. Temperature changes, humidity fluctuations, air quality issues, and even subtle chemical exposures can trigger or worsen nocturnal episodes.

Temperature Sensitivity During Vulnerable Hours: Many MCAS patients report that temperature changes during the night trigger episodes. This might be cooling from air conditioning, warming from heating systems cycling on, or even the natural temperature drop that occurs during deep sleep. The key is maintaining stable temperatures during the 1-5am window.

Air Quality Management: Indoor air quality often deteriorates overnight as HVAC systems cycle less frequently and outdoor pollutants accumulate. HEPA filtration systems should run continuously during nighttime hours, and bedroom doors should be kept closed to maintain clean air zones.

Chemical Sensitivity Peaks: The same circadian factors that make mast cells more reactive also make them more sensitive to chemical triggers. Fragrances, cleaning products, or off-gassing from furniture and bedding that might be tolerable during the day can trigger episodes during vulnerable hours.

Pre-emptive Strike Strategies

Evening Medication Protocols

The most effective approach to managing 2-4am episodes is preventing them entirely through strategic evening medication timing. This isn't about taking more medications — it's about taking the right medications at the right times to provide protection during vulnerable hours.

Standard Evening Protocol:

- **10:00 PM:** Mast cell stabilizers (quercetin 500mg, cromolyn sodium if prescribed)
- **10:30 PM:** H2 antihistamine (famotidine 20mg or ranitidine if available)
- **11:00 PM:** H1 antihistamine (cetirizine 10mg or loratadine 10mg for long-acting coverage)
- **11:30 PM:** Additional H1 if needed (diphenhydramine 25mg for severe symptoms)

Advanced Evening Protocol for Severe Cases:

- **9:30 PM:** Natural mast cell stabilizers (quercetin with bromelain)
- **10:00 PM:** Prescription mast cell stabilizers (ketotifen if prescribed)
- **10:30 PM:** H2 antihistamine with proton pump inhibitor if needed
- **11:00 PM:** Combination H1 antihistamine (cetirizine + loratadine)
- **11:30 PM:** Low-dose melatonin (0.5mg) if tolerated

- **12:00 AM:** Additional H1 if breakthrough symptoms anticipated

Individual Customization: The exact timing and medication choices need individualization based on your specific pattern of episodes. Some patients have earlier episodes (midnight-2am) requiring earlier medication timing. Others have later episodes (4-6am) allowing for later medication administration.

Supplement Timing for Maximum Effect

Natural supplements can provide significant benefit for nocturnal histamine surges, but timing is critical for effectiveness. Many patients take supplements randomly throughout the day without considering when they need maximum protection.

Quercetin Optimization: Quercetin is most effective when taken with bromelain and vitamin C to enhance absorption. The optimal timing for nocturnal protection is 2-3 hours before anticipated symptoms, typically around 10pm-11pm. Taking quercetin with a small amount of fat (like a few nuts) can improve absorption significantly.

Magnesium for Nervous System Calming: Magnesium glycinate or magnesium taurate taken 1-2 hours before bed can help modulate the stress response that triggers mast cell activation. The goal isn't sedation — it's nervous system stabilization during vulnerable hours.

Vitamin C as Natural Antihistamine: Vitamin C has natural antihistamine properties and can help stabilize mast cell membranes. Time-release vitamin C taken around 10pm provides sustained levels during overnight hours. Typical doses range from 500-1000mg depending on tolerance.

B-Complex for Histamine Metabolism: B vitamins, particularly B6 and B12, support histamine metabolism pathways. Taking a B-complex supplement with dinner (around 6pm) ensures adequate cofactors are available during overnight histamine processing.

Bedroom Environment Optimization

Your bedroom environment becomes critically important during the vulnerable 2-4am window. Small environmental factors that might not matter during the day can trigger or worsen episodes during this sensitive time period.

Temperature Control Strategies: Maintain bedroom temperature between 65-68°F (18-20°C) during nighttime hours. Avoid significant temperature fluctuations from heating or cooling systems cycling on and off. Some patients benefit from programmable thermostats that maintain very stable temperatures during the 1-5am window.

Humidity Management: Indoor humidity should be maintained between 40-50% to minimize mold growth while preventing excessive dryness that can irritate airways and skin. Humidifiers or dehumidifiers should run quietly to avoid sleep disruption while maintaining optimal levels.

Air Filtration Systems: HEPA air purifiers should run continuously during nighttime hours, not on timer settings. The goal is maintaining consistently clean air during vulnerable hours. Position air purifiers to create gentle air circulation without creating drafts that might trigger temperature sensitivity.

Chemical Exposure Minimization: Use only fragrance-free, hypoallergenic bedding and pajamas. Wash all bedding in fragrance-free detergent and avoid fabric softeners. Keep bedroom doors closed during sleeping hours to maintain a clean air zone separate from the rest of the house.

Dietary Considerations for Histamine Management

The timing of your last meal and the histamine content of evening foods can significantly impact nocturnal symptoms. High-histamine foods consumed late in the day can contribute to overall histamine load during vulnerable overnight hours.

Evening Meal Timing: Finish eating at least 3-4 hours before your typical episode time. For most patients, this means finishing dinner by 6pm-7pm if episodes typically occur around 2-4am. Late eating can trigger gastric acid production and digestive processes that may worsen mast cell reactivity.

Low-Histamine Evening Food Choices:

- Fresh proteins (chicken, fish, turkey) prepared simply
- Fresh vegetables (avoid tomatoes, spinach, eggplant)
- Rice, quinoa, or other non-fermented grains
- Fresh fruits (avoid citrus, strawberries, bananas)
- Herbal teas (chamomile, ginger) instead of alcohol or caffeine

Foods to Avoid in Evening Hours:

- Fermented foods (wine, cheese, yogurt, sauerkraut)
- Aged or processed meats (salami, pepperoni, hot dogs)
- Leftover foods (histamine increases with storage time)
- Citrus fruits and tomatoes
- Chocolate and caffeinated beverages
- Alcohol of any type

Active Crisis Management

Immediate Intervention Protocols

Despite best prevention efforts, breakthrough episodes still occur. Having a systematic approach to managing active episodes can minimize their severity and duration. The key is rapid, targeted intervention that addresses multiple pathways simultaneously.

First 15 Minutes Protocol:

1. **Immediate positioning:** Sit up or elevate head of bed to 30-45 degrees
2. **Fast-acting antihistamine:** Liquid diphenhydramine 25-50mg
3. **H2 blocker:** Famotidine 20mg if you can swallow

4. **Cooling measures:** Cool compress to neck, wrists, or chest
5. **Breathing support:** Slow, controlled breathing to prevent hyperventilation

Next 15-30 Minutes:

1. **Additional antihistamines:** Second H1 antihistamine if symptoms persist
2. **Mast cell stabilizers:** Quercetin or cromolyn if not already taken
3. **Hydration:** Cool water with electrolytes, avoiding histamine-rich beverages
4. **Environmental adjustments:** Ensure optimal room temperature and air circulation
5. **Symptom monitoring:** Track heart rate, blood pressure if available, overall symptom severity

30-60 Minutes Post-Episode:

1. **Sustained antihistamine coverage:** Long-acting H1 if breakthrough occurred
2. **Recovery positioning:** Maintain elevated position until symptoms fully resolve
3. **Gentle rehydration:** Continue fluid replacement with electrolyte balance
4. **Sleep position optimization:** Adjust pillows and supports for comfortable return to sleep
5. **Documentation:** Record episode details for pattern recognition

Symptom-Specific Treatment Approaches

Different patients experience different manifestations of nocturnal histamine surges, and treatment should be tailored to predominant symptoms while addressing the underlying mast cell activation.

Cardiovascular Symptoms (Tachycardia, Palpitations):

- Immediate vagal maneuvers (bearing down, cold water on face)
- Electrolyte replacement (magnesium, potassium)
- Beta-blocker if prescribed for breakthrough episodes
- Position changes to optimize venous return
- Continuous heart rate monitoring if equipment available

Respiratory Symptoms (Wheezing, Throat Tightness):

- Albuterol inhaler for bronchospasm
- Cool mist to reduce airway inflammation
- Elevated positioning to improve lung expansion
- Controlled breathing techniques to prevent hyperventilation
- Emergency epinephrine if severe throat swelling occurs

Gastrointestinal Symptoms (Nausea, Cramping, Diarrhea):

- H2 antihistamines for gastric acid control
- Simethicone for gas and bloating
- Small sips of clear fluids to prevent dehydration
- Avoid solid foods until symptoms resolve
- Probiotics the following day to restore gut balance

Neurological Symptoms (Anxiety, Panic, Cognitive Fog):

- Grounding techniques to manage anxiety
- Cool compress to forehead and neck
- Magnesium supplementation for nervous system support
- Avoid stimulating activities or bright lights
- Focus on slow, deep breathing to activate parasympathetic response

Recovery Techniques and Sleep Restoration

Getting back to sleep after a nocturnal histamine surge can be challenging because your nervous system remains activated even after histamine levels decrease. Specific techniques can help facilitate the transition back to restorative sleep.

Nervous System Reset Protocol:

1. **Progressive muscle relaxation:** Systematically tense and release muscle groups
2. **Guided imagery:** Focus on calming scenes or sensations
3. **Breathing exercises:** 4-7-8 breathing pattern or box breathing
4. **Meditation techniques:** Body scanning or mindfulness practices
5. **Temperature regulation:** Ensure optimal comfort for sleep return

Sleep Environment Restoration:

- Check and adjust room temperature if needed
- Ensure bedding hasn't become uncomfortable from sweating
- Adjust pillows and supports for optimal positioning
- Minimize light exposure to preserve melatonin
- Use white noise or earplugs if environmental sounds are bothersome

Medication Considerations for Sleep Return:

- Avoid stimulating medications that might prevent sleep return
- Consider low-dose melatonin (0.5mg) if episode occurs before 3am
- Magnesium supplementation can help with muscle relaxation
- Avoid caffeine or other stimulants even if you feel tired
- Time any additional medications to avoid morning drowsiness

Documentation for Pattern Recognition

Systematic documentation of nocturnal episodes is essential for identifying triggers, assessing treatment effectiveness, and communicating with healthcare providers. Most patients underestimate the value of detailed record-keeping until they start seeing patterns.

Essential Documentation Elements:

- **Exact timing:** When did symptoms begin, peak, and resolve?
- **Symptom details:** What symptoms occurred and in what order?
- **Trigger assessment:** What might have contributed to this episode?
- **Treatment response:** What interventions were used and how effective were they?
- **Recovery time:** How long until normal sleep could resume?

Pattern Recognition Analysis:

- **Weekly patterns:** Do episodes occur more frequently on certain days?
- **Monthly patterns:** Is there correlation with menstrual cycles?
- **Seasonal patterns:** Do episodes worsen during certain times of year?
- **Environmental correlations:** Are episodes associated with weather, allergens, or chemical exposures?
- **Dietary correlations:** Do certain foods or meal timing patterns correlate with episodes?

Treatment Optimization Data:

- **Medication effectiveness:** Which interventions provide the most reliable relief?
- **Timing optimization:** What medication timing provides the best prevention?
- **Dose adjustments:** Do you need higher or lower doses of specific medications?
- **Environmental modifications:** Which environmental changes provide the most benefit?
- **Lifestyle factors:** How do sleep schedule, stress, and activity levels affect episode frequency?

Real-World Application Challenges

The biggest challenge with 2-4am crisis management is implementing protocols when you're half-awake, potentially scared, and dealing with physical symptoms that affect your thinking clearly. This is why preparation and practice are so important — your crisis protocol needs to be simple enough to follow when you're not at your best.

Many patients resist taking evening medications because they worry about side effects or drug interactions. But the reality is that preventing episodes is much safer and more effective than trying to treat them after they've started. The medications used for prevention are generally well-tolerated and much less problematic than dealing with repeated nocturnal crises.

The documentation aspect often gets neglected because patients are too tired or overwhelmed during and after episodes. But this information is critically important for optimizing your prevention and treatment strategies. Consider keeping a simple voice recorder or smartphone app that allows quick recording of episode details without having to write extensively.

The Path to Peaceful Nights

Managing the 2-4am crisis pattern requires a shift from reactive to proactive thinking. Instead of waiting for episodes to occur and then trying to treat them, the goal is preventing them entirely through strategic timing of interventions and environmental optimization.

This approach takes time to implement and refine, but most patients see significant improvement within 2-4 weeks of consistent application. The key is being systematic about medication timing, environmental control, and documentation while being patient with the process of finding your optimal protocol.

The next chapter will address the broader topic of temperature regulation, because the temperature sensitivity that often accompanies mast cell episodes is a major factor in sleep disruption that extends well beyond the 2-4am window.

Crisis Management Essentials:

- Implement pre-emptive evening medication protocols timed to provide maximum protection during the vulnerable 2-4am window
- Optimize bedroom environment for temperature stability, air quality, and chemical sensitivity management
- Develop systematic crisis intervention protocols that address multiple symptom types rapidly and effectively
- Maintain detailed documentation of episodes to identify patterns and optimize prevention strategies
- Focus on sleep restoration techniques that help facilitate return to restorative sleep after episodes
- Recognize that prevention is more effective and safer than treatment of active episodes

Chapter 6: Advanced Temperature Dysregulation Management

Your body's temperature control system isn't just broken — it's been sabotaged by conditions that turn your internal thermostat into something resembling a malfunctioning carnival ride. One minute you're freezing cold despite being under three blankets, the next you're sweating through your sheets from some invisible heat source that has nothing to do with room temperature. This isn't just uncomfortable; it's physiologically disruptive to sleep architecture and can trigger symptom cascades that keep you awake for hours.

The temperature regulation problems in EDS, POTS, and MCAS aren't minor inconveniences that you can solve with a fan or an extra blanket. They're manifestations of serious dysfunction in autonomic nervous system control, mast cell reactivity, and connective tissue properties that require sophisticated management strategies. Understanding these mechanisms isn't academic — it's the foundation for developing interventions that actually work.

Understanding Your Internal Thermostat

Sudomotor Dysfunction Mechanisms

Sweating isn't just about cooling off — it's a complex process controlled by the sympathetic nervous system that involves precise coordination between nerve signals, sweat gland function, and blood vessel responses. In POTS patients, this entire system is compromised, leading to inappropriate sweating, lack of sweating when needed, and temperature regulation that seems completely disconnected from environmental conditions.

The sympathetic nerves that control sweating (sudomotor function) are often damaged or dysfunctional in POTS patients. Research shows that up to 70% of POTS patients have evidence of sudomotor dysfunction on specialized testing, but most patients and even many doctors don't recognize this as part of the condition (Thieben et al., 2007). This dysfunction manifests as either excessive sweating (hyperhidrosis) or inadequate sweating (anhidrosis), often in patterns that make no physiological sense.

Distal vs. Proximal Sweating Patterns: Many POTS patients develop abnormal sweating patterns where their hands and feet sweat excessively while their trunk and back don't sweat adequately. This creates a situation where you feel simultaneously clammy and overheated, making temperature regulation nearly impossible. During sleep, this can mean waking up with soaking wet hands and feet while your core temperature remains elevated.

Gustatory Sweating: Some patients develop gustatory sweating — excessive sweating triggered by eating certain foods or even thinking about food. This can be particularly problematic if it occurs after evening meals, creating temperature regulation problems just as you're trying to prepare for sleep.

Exercise Intolerance and Heat Buildup: The inability to sweat appropriately means that even minimal physical activity can cause dangerous heat buildup. For sleep preparation, this means that normal evening activities like showering or light stretching can trigger overheating that persists for hours, making sleep onset nearly impossible.

Vasomotor Instability Patterns

Blood vessel control is fundamental to temperature regulation, and the autonomic dysfunction in POTS creates chaotic patterns of blood vessel constriction and dilation that make stable temperature control impossible. Your blood vessels are supposed to dilate when you need cooling and constrict when you need warming, but in POTS, they often do the opposite or change inappropriately in response to minor stimuli.

Peripheral Vasodilation Problems: Normal cooling involves dilation of blood vessels in the hands, feet, and skin surface to allow heat

63

dissipation. In POTS patients, this mechanism often fails, leading to heat retention even when environmental temperatures are cool. During sleep, this manifests as feeling overheated regardless of room temperature or bedding choices.

Raynaud's-like Phenomena: Many POTS patients experience Raynaud's-like symptoms where hands and feet become extremely cold and may change colors. This can occur even in warm environments and can be triggered by minor stress or position changes. During sleep, this creates the bizarre situation of having cold extremities while feeling overheated centrally.

Postural Blood Flow Changes: Position changes that are normal during sleep can trigger dramatic blood vessel responses in POTS patients. Rolling from side to back might trigger flushing and overheating, while lying flat might cause blood pooling that makes you feel cold and clammy. These position-triggered temperature changes can wake you up repeatedly throughout the night.

MCAS-Related Temperature Fluctuations

Mast cell mediators have direct effects on blood vessels and temperature regulation that can override normal physiological controls. Histamine, in particular, is a potent vasodilator that can trigger sudden flushing and overheating episodes. But mast cells also release other mediators that can cause paradoxical cooling or temperature instability that seems unrelated to environmental factors.

Histamine-Induced Vasodilation: When mast cells degranulate, the released histamine causes immediate vasodilation, particularly in skin blood vessels. This creates the characteristic flushing seen in mast cell reactions, but it also disrupts normal temperature control. During sleep, even minor mast cell activation can trigger flushing episodes that wake you up feeling overheated and uncomfortable.

Prostaglandin Effects: Mast cells also release prostaglandins, which have complex effects on temperature regulation. Some prostaglandins cause fever-like responses, while others can cause hypothermia-like cooling. The net effect is often temperature instability that fluctuates unpredictably and doesn't respond to environmental temperature changes.

Leukotriene-Mediated Responses: Leukotrienes released during mast cell activation can cause blood vessel constriction in some areas while causing dilation in others. This creates chaotic temperature regulation where different parts of your body may feel hot or cold simultaneously, making it impossible to find comfortable sleeping conditions.

Individual Variation Assessment

The temperature regulation problems in these conditions vary dramatically between individuals, and effective management requires understanding your specific patterns. Some patients are primarily heat-intolerant, others are cold-intolerant, and many fluctuate unpredictably between both extremes.

Heat-Predominant Patterns:

- Excessive sweating with minimal activity
- Feeling overheated in normal room temperatures
- Difficulty cooling down after becoming warm
- Night sweats unrelated to environmental temperature
- Flushing episodes triggered by stress, food, or medications

Cold-Predominant Patterns:

- Feeling cold even in warm environments
- Extremities that remain cold regardless of core temperature
- Difficulty warming up once cold
- Shivering or feeling chilled during normal activities
- Cold sensitivity that seems out of proportion to temperature

Mixed or Fluctuating Patterns:

- Alternating between feeling too hot and too cold

- Different body parts at different temperatures simultaneously
- Temperature sensitivity that changes based on time of day or activity level
- Unpredictable responses to environmental temperature changes
- Temperature regulation that seems disconnected from actual ambient temperature

Evidence-Based Cooling Strategies

Medical-Grade Cooling Systems

Standard fans and air conditioning often aren't sufficient for patients with severe temperature regulation dysfunction. Medical-grade cooling systems provide more precise temperature control and can be targeted to specific body areas that need cooling while avoiding overcooling of sensitive areas.

Cooling Vest Technology: Medical cooling vests use phase-change materials or circulating cool water to provide sustained cooling without the bulk and discomfort of ice packs. These systems can be particularly useful for patients who experience overheating during sleep preparation activities or who need cooling support during the night.

Mattress Cooling Systems: Specialized mattress cooling systems circulate temperature-controlled water through thin tubes embedded in mattress pads. These systems allow precise temperature control (often adjustable to within 1-2 degrees) and can be set to different temperatures for different parts of the bed. Some systems allow independent temperature control for each side of the bed, which is useful when partners have different temperature needs.

Targeted Cooling Devices: Cooling devices that target specific body areas (neck, wrists, temples) can be more effective than whole-body cooling for some patients. These areas have blood vessels close to the skin surface, and cooling them can help reduce overall body temperature more efficiently than general environmental cooling.

Strategic Timing of Interventions

The timing of cooling interventions is often as important as the interventions themselves. Understanding your body's natural temperature rhythms and how they're disrupted by your conditions allows for strategic cooling that prevents overheating rather than trying to treat it after it occurs.

Pre-Sleep Cooling Protocols: Begin cooling interventions 2-3 hours before bedtime to allow your body temperature to reach optimal levels for sleep onset. Normal physiology requires a drop in core body temperature for sleep initiation, and patients with temperature regulation dysfunction often need help achieving this drop.

Circadian Temperature Management: Body temperature normally peaks in late afternoon/early evening and reaches its lowest point around 4-6am. Patients with autonomic dysfunction often have disrupted circadian temperature rhythms that require external support to maintain normal patterns.

Activity-Based Cooling: Plan cooling interventions around activities that tend to trigger overheating. This might mean pre-cooling before showers, meals, or any physical activity that typically causes temperature dysregulation.

Hydration and Electrolyte Protocols

Temperature regulation is intimately connected to hydration status and electrolyte balance. Dehydration impairs sweating ability, while electrolyte imbalances can affect blood vessel function and temperature control mechanisms.

Strategic Hydration Timing: Hydration for temperature regulation isn't just about drinking water — it's about maintaining optimal blood volume and electrolyte balance throughout the day. For sleep preparation, this means ensuring adequate hydration 2-3 hours before bedtime while avoiding excessive fluids that might cause nighttime urination.

Electrolyte Optimization: Sodium, potassium, and magnesium all play roles in blood vessel function and temperature regulation. Many POTS patients require higher sodium intake (3-10 grams per day), but this needs to be balanced with adequate potassium and magnesium to prevent muscle cramping and maintain optimal blood vessel function.

Temperature-Specific Hydration: Use cool (not ice-cold) fluids for internal cooling when overheated. Ice-cold beverages can actually trigger vasoconstriction that impairs heat dissipation. Room temperature or slightly cool fluids are more effective for cooling purposes.

Managing Cold Intolerance

Layered Warming Strategies

Cold intolerance in these conditions isn't just about environmental temperature — it often reflects impaired circulation, autonomic dysfunction, or metabolic issues that require targeted warming strategies rather than simply adding more blankets.

Progressive Warming Systems: Instead of trying to warm up quickly (which can trigger inappropriate autonomic responses), use progressive warming that gradually increases body temperature. This might involve starting with light warming and gradually adding layers or heat sources as tolerated.

Targeted Warming Zones: Focus warming efforts on areas that tend to get coldest first — typically hands, feet, and sometimes the core. Warming these areas can help improve overall circulation and temperature regulation more effectively than general environmental warming.

Circulation Enhancement: Cold intolerance often reflects poor circulation rather than just environmental cold. Light movement, gentle massage, or positioning changes can help improve blood flow to cold areas more effectively than passive warming alone.

Compression Garment Integration

Compression garments can help with both temperature regulation and circulation improvement, but they need to be used strategically to avoid creating additional problems.

Temperature-Appropriate Compression: Choose compression garments made from materials that provide appropriate temperature regulation. Some materials trap heat (useful for cold intolerance), while others wick moisture and provide cooling (useful for heat intolerance).

Graduated Compression Benefits: Properly fitted graduated compression stockings can improve circulation to the extremities, helping address the cold hands and feet that many patients experience. The improved circulation often helps with overall temperature regulation, not just warming of the compressed areas.

Sleep-Safe Compression: Not all compression garments are appropriate for nighttime use. Choose garments specifically designed for extended wear that won't restrict circulation if you move during sleep or if swelling patterns change overnight.

Seasonal Adaptation Protocols

Temperature regulation problems often worsen during seasonal transitions or extreme weather, requiring adaptive strategies that change based on environmental conditions and seasonal physiological changes.

Winter Adaptation Strategies:

- Gradual indoor temperature increases rather than dramatic heating
- Humidity management to prevent dry air from worsening symptoms
- Light therapy to support circadian rhythms during dark months

- Vitamin D supplementation to support immune and autonomic function
- Strategic timing of outdoor activities to minimize cold exposure stress

Summer Adaptation Strategies:

- Gradual acclimatization to higher temperatures over several weeks
- Pre-cooling before going outdoors in hot weather
- Strategic timing of activities during cooler parts of the day
- Enhanced hydration and electrolyte replacement during hot weather
- Environmental modifications to maintain cool indoor spaces

Transition Season Management: Spring and fall can be particularly challenging because of rapid temperature fluctuations that stress already-compromised temperature regulation systems. During these seasons, focus on having multiple layers available and being prepared for rapid temperature changes throughout the day.

Creating the Optimal Sleep Environment

Zone-Specific Climate Management

Your bedroom needs to become a carefully controlled environment that supports stable temperature regulation throughout the night. This often requires more sophisticated climate control than a simple thermostat adjustment.

Micro-Climate Creation: Use combinations of heating and cooling devices to create different temperature zones within your bedroom. You might need cooling for your upper body while requiring warmth for your feet, or you might need different temperatures at different times during the night.

Humidity Control Integration: Temperature and humidity work together to create comfort. Low humidity can make you feel colder than the actual temperature, while high humidity can make you feel overheated. Optimal bedroom humidity is typically 40-50%, but some patients need more precise control based on their specific sensitivities.

Air Circulation Management: Moving air can help with cooling, but it can also create drafts that trigger cold sensitivity. Use ceiling fans on low settings or strategically placed fans to create gentle air circulation without creating uncomfortable drafts.

HEPA Filtration and Air Quality

Air quality affects both respiratory function and temperature regulation. Poor air quality can trigger mast cell reactions that disrupt temperature control, while good air quality supports optimal sleep and temperature regulation.

Continuous Filtration: Run HEPA air purifiers continuously during sleeping hours, not just during the day. Nighttime air quality is often worse due to reduced air circulation and accumulation of indoor pollutants.

Filter Maintenance: Replace HEPA filters regularly — dirty filters reduce effectiveness and can actually worsen air quality. Check filters monthly and replace according to manufacturer recommendations or sooner if you live in areas with high pollution or allergen levels.

Chemical Filtration: Some patients benefit from air purifiers that include activated carbon filters to remove chemical odors and volatile organic compounds that might trigger temperature regulation problems or mast cell reactions.

The Temperature Regulation Reality Check

Temperature regulation problems in EDS, POTS, and MCAS aren't quirky personal preferences or minor inconveniences — they're serious physiological dysfunctions that require systematic management approaches. Dismissing these problems as "just being sensitive to temperature" misses the underlying autonomic and inflammatory mechanisms that need targeted intervention.

The most frustrating aspect is how often these problems are minimized by healthcare providers who don't understand the complexity of temperature regulation dysfunction in these conditions. Patients aren't being dramatic or difficult when they report temperature problems — they're describing real physiological dysfunction that significantly impacts their quality of life and sleep quality.

Effective temperature regulation management requires patience, experimentation, and often significant investment in environmental control systems. But the payoff in terms of improved sleep quality and overall symptom management makes this investment worthwhile for most patients.

The next chapter will expand on environmental optimization beyond just temperature control, addressing the broader sensory and chemical factors that can make or break your sleep environment.

Temperature Management Mastery Points:

- Recognize temperature regulation problems as serious physiological dysfunction requiring systematic management, not simple environmental adjustments
- Implement both cooling and warming strategies based on your individual patterns of temperature dysregulation
- Use medical-grade temperature control systems when standard environmental controls are insufficient
- Integrate hydration and electrolyte management as part of temperature regulation protocols
- Create bedroom micro-climates that address your specific temperature regulation needs throughout the night
- Adapt temperature management strategies seasonally and based on changing environmental conditions

Chapter 7: Creating the Optimal Sleep Environment

Your bedroom isn't just where you sleep — it's a complex sensory environment that can either support or sabotage your attempts at restorative sleep. For patients with EDS, POTS, and MCAS, this environment becomes critically important because your heightened sensitivities mean that factors barely noticeable to healthy individuals can trigger hours of sleep disruption. Creating an optimal sleep environment isn't about buying expensive gadgets; it's about systematically addressing the sensory, chemical, and physical factors that interfere with sleep in sensitive individuals.

Most sleep hygiene advice assumes you have normal sensory processing and average sensitivity to environmental factors. That advice is useless for patients whose mast cells react to trace chemical exposures, whose autonomic systems are triggered by minor light or sound changes, and whose hypermobile joints require specific positioning support. You need an approach that acknowledges your unique physiological challenges and addresses them systematically.

Temperature and Humidity Control

Zone-Specific Climate Management

Creating optimal sleep conditions often requires more sophisticated climate control than a single thermostat can provide. Your head might need cooling while your feet need warming, or you might need different temperatures at different times throughout the night as your symptoms fluctuate.

Dual-Zone Temperature Systems: Many patients benefit from mattress systems that allow independent temperature control for different areas of the bed. The head zone might be set to 65°F while the foot zone is set to 70°F, accommodating the circulation problems common in POTS and the temperature sensitivity patterns seen in MCAS.

Vertical Temperature Gradients: Room temperature at floor level is often 5-10 degrees cooler than at ceiling level. Use this natural gradient strategically — if you tend to run hot, position your bed lower in the room and use floor-level cooling. If you tend to run cold, elevate your bed slightly and use ceiling fans to circulate warmer air downward.

Temporal Temperature Control: Program your climate control systems to accommodate your circadian temperature needs. Many patients need cooler temperatures during the 2-4am histamine surge period, then slightly warmer temperatures during the 4-6am period when core body temperature naturally reaches its lowest point.

Micro-Climate Creation Tools:

- Bedside fans for targeted air circulation
- Heating pads designed for extended use
- Cooling mattress toppers with temperature control
- Weighted blankets that provide warmth without overheating
- Breathable bed linens that wick moisture while maintaining temperature

HEPA Filtration and Air Quality Management

Air quality becomes critically important for patients whose mast cells react to airborne triggers and whose respiratory systems are sensitive to irritants. Poor air quality doesn't just affect breathing — it can trigger cascades of symptoms that disrupt sleep for hours.

Continuous HEPA Filtration: Standard air conditioning filters aren't sufficient for sensitive patients. True HEPA filters remove 99.97% of particles 0.3 microns or larger, including dust mites, pollen, pet dander, and many chemical particles. Run HEPA purifiers continuously during sleeping hours, positioned to create clean air circulation around your bed.

Filter Sizing and Placement: Choose HEPA purifiers rated for rooms larger than your actual bedroom to ensure adequate air turnover. Position units to create air circulation patterns that draw contaminated air away from your bed while providing clean air circulation around your sleeping area.

Multi-Stage Filtration: Many patients benefit from air purifiers that combine HEPA filtration with activated carbon filters to remove volatile organic compounds and chemical odors. Some units also include UV germicidal lights to eliminate bacteria and viruses, though these should be used cautiously as some patients are sensitive to UV exposure.

Maintenance Protocols:

- Replace pre-filters monthly during high-allergen seasons
- Replace HEPA filters every 6-12 months or according to air quality monitor readings
- Clean air purifier exteriors weekly to prevent dust accumulation
- Monitor air quality with indoor air quality meters to track filtration effectiveness

Hypoallergenic Material Selection

The materials in your bedroom environment can be significant sources of allergens, irritants, and chemical exposures that disrupt sleep. This goes beyond just having "allergy-friendly" bedding — it requires systematic evaluation of every material that might affect your air quality or trigger sensitivities.

Bedding Material Optimization: Natural materials aren't automatically better for sensitive patients. Organic cotton can harbor dust mites, wool can trigger reactions in sensitive individuals, and down can be a major allergen source. Synthetic materials designed for allergen control often provide better results than natural alternatives.

Recommended Bedding Materials:

- Tightly woven synthetic fabrics that prevent dust mite penetration
- Bamboo-derived fabrics that naturally resist bacteria and mold
- Specially treated cotton that has been processed to remove natural allergens
- Memory foam pillows and mattress toppers with hypoallergenic covers
- Silk, which naturally resists dust mites and is often well-tolerated

Furniture and Flooring Considerations: Upholstered furniture in bedrooms can harbor allergens and chemicals that off-gas during nighttime hours. Hard flooring surfaces are generally better than carpeting for sensitive patients, but area rugs that can be frequently washed may provide comfort without creating allergen reservoirs.

Chemical and Fragrance Elimination

Chemical sensitivities in MCAS patients can be triggered by exposures so minimal that they're undetectable to most people. Creating a chemically clean sleep environment requires attention to sources of chemical exposure that most people never consider.

Cleaning Product Protocols: Use only fragrance-free, dye-free cleaning products in bedroom areas. Many patients find that even "natural" or "green" cleaning products contain essential oils or plant-based chemicals that trigger reactions. Simple solutions like white vinegar, baking soda, and unscented soap often work better than commercial products.

Off-Gassing Management: New furniture, mattresses, and even bedding can off-gas chemicals for weeks or months. When possible, air out new items in non-bedroom areas before bringing them into your sleep environment. Some patients need to wrap new mattresses in aluminum barriers and allow several weeks of off-gassing before use.

Personal Care Product Timing: Evening skincare routines, hair products, and even toothpaste can introduce chemicals into your sleep environment. Use fragrance-free products and complete your evening routine at least 30 minutes before entering your bedroom to allow chemical dissipation.

Hidden Chemical Sources:

- Fabric softeners and dryer sheets (residues persist on clothing and bedding)
- Scented laundry detergents (can off-gas from clothing in closets)
- Room deodorizers and air fresheners (including "natural" essential oil diffusers)
- Insect control products (sprays, plug-ins, treated materials)
- Electronic equipment (some plastics and components off-gas chemicals)

Sensory Considerations

Light Management for Circadian Support

Light exposure during evening and nighttime hours is one of the most powerful disruptors of circadian rhythms and sleep quality. For patients with autonomic dysfunction, proper light management becomes even more critical because disrupted circadian rhythms can worsen POTS symptoms and trigger mast cell reactivity.

Blue Light Elimination: Blue light from electronic devices, LED bulbs, and even some fluorescent lights can suppress melatonin production and disrupt circadian rhythms. Begin blue light elimination 2-3 hours before bedtime using blue light blocking glasses, screen filters, or apps that adjust device color temperature.

Evening Light Protocols:

- Use warm-colored lights (2700K or lower) in bedroom areas after sunset
- Install dimmer switches to gradually reduce light intensity as bedtime approaches

- Use red or amber night lights for nighttime navigation (these don't disrupt melatonin)
- Consider blackout curtains or eye masks to eliminate all light during sleep hours
- Position alarm clocks and electronic devices so displays don't create light pollution

Morning Light Therapy: Appropriate morning light exposure helps maintain healthy circadian rhythms and can improve nighttime sleep quality. For POTS patients who have difficulty with morning activities, light therapy boxes can provide circadian support without requiring outdoor exposure during symptom-heavy morning hours.

Sound Dampening for Hypervigilance

Many patients with these conditions develop hypervigilance — an increased alertness to environmental threats that makes it difficult to relax and fall asleep. Sound dampening isn't just about blocking loud noises; it's about creating a predictable auditory environment that doesn't trigger alertness responses.

White Noise vs. Pink Noise: White noise contains all frequencies at equal intensity and can help mask disruptive sounds. Pink noise has more low-frequency content and is often more soothing for sleep. Some patients prefer brown noise, which has even more low-frequency emphasis and can feel more like natural environmental sounds.

Sound Masking Strategies:

- Continuous background noise helps mask intermittent sounds that might wake you
- Fan noise provides consistent sound masking while also creating air circulation
- Dedicated white noise machines often provide better sound quality than phone apps
- Earplugs designed for sleeping can reduce overall noise levels without complete sound elimination

- Strategic room arrangement can help minimize noise transmission from other areas

Hypervigilance Management: Patients with chronic illness often develop heightened alertness to potential threats, making it difficult to achieve the relaxed state necessary for sleep onset. Sound management needs to account for this psychological component, not just physical noise reduction.

Texture Selection for Proprioceptive Comfort

Patients with EDS often have altered proprioception and sensory processing that makes certain textures uncomfortable or disruptive to sleep. The goal is finding materials that provide appropriate sensory input without creating irritation or distraction.

Fabric Texture Considerations: Smooth, cool fabrics like bamboo or silk often work well for patients with skin sensitivity. Avoid rough textures, scratchy seams, or materials that create static electricity. Some patients prefer the deep pressure sensation of weighted blankets, while others find any weight intolerable.

Mattress Surface Optimization: Memory foam provides pressure relief for sensitive joints but can retain heat and make position changes difficult. Latex provides more responsiveness but may be too firm for some patients. Hybrid mattresses that combine different materials often provide the best compromise between support and comfort.

Pillow Engineering: Pillow selection affects both comfort and joint stability. The goal is providing support that maintains proper spinal alignment while accommodating individual joint stability needs and texture preferences.

Scent-Free Protocols for MCAS

Chemical sensitivities in MCAS patients extend to natural fragrances, essential oils, and even the subtle scents from personal care products and laundry treatments. Creating a truly scent-free environment requires attention to sources of fragrance that most people don't even notice.

Complete Fragrance Elimination:

- Use only fragrance-free and dye-free laundry products
- Avoid fabric softeners and dryer sheets entirely
- Choose personal care products labeled "fragrance-free" rather than "unscented" (unscented products may contain masking fragrances)
- Eliminate air fresheners, candles, and essential oil diffusers from bedroom areas
- Be aware that "natural" products often contain plant-based fragrances that can trigger reactions

Partner Cooperation: If you share a bedroom, your partner's personal care products can affect your air quality. This often requires compromise and cooperation to maintain a scent-free environment that supports your health needs while respecting your partner's preferences.

Visitor Protocols: Guests may inadvertently introduce fragrances through their clothing, personal care products, or belongings. Having polite but clear guidelines about fragrance-free visiting can help maintain your sleep environment when others are in your home.

Implementation and Maintenance

Systematic Environmental Assessment

Creating an optimal sleep environment requires systematic evaluation of all environmental factors rather than making random changes and hoping for improvement. Start with a baseline assessment of your current environment and systematically address each factor that might be affecting your sleep quality.

Environmental Audit Protocol: Spend several nights documenting your current sleep environment and any factors that seem to correlate with sleep disruption. Note temperature fluctuations, noise sources, light pollution, chemical exposures, and comfort issues. This baseline assessment helps prioritize which environmental modifications will provide the greatest benefit.

Gradual Implementation Strategy: Making multiple environmental changes simultaneously makes it impossible to determine which modifications are helpful and which might be problematic. Implement changes one at a time over several weeks, allowing adequate time to assess the impact of each modification before adding new elements.

Cost-Effective Prioritization: Environmental modifications can become expensive quickly. Prioritize changes based on their potential impact and cost-effectiveness. Simple modifications like eliminating fragrances and improving air circulation often provide significant benefits at minimal cost, while expensive equipment purchases should be reserved for issues that can't be addressed through simpler means.

Maintenance and Monitoring Protocols

An optimal sleep environment requires ongoing maintenance to remain effective. Environmental factors change seasonally, equipment needs regular servicing, and your sensitivities may evolve over time, requiring adjustments to your environmental protocols.

Regular Maintenance Schedules:

- Weekly: Wash bedding in fragrance-free detergent, clean air purifier exterior surfaces, assess room for new chemical exposures
- Monthly: Replace air purifier pre-filters, check HEPA filter condition, evaluate temperature and humidity control effectiveness
- Seasonally: Replace HEPA filters, assess clothing and bedding for wear or allergen accumulation, adjust environmental controls for seasonal changes
- Annually: Professional HVAC cleaning and maintenance, mattress and pillow replacement assessment, comprehensive environmental audit

Environmental Monitoring Tools: Consider investing in indoor air quality monitors that track temperature, humidity, particulate matter, and volatile organic compounds. These devices provide objective data about your sleep environment and can help identify problems before they significantly impact your sleep quality.

Adaptation and Optimization: Your environmental needs may change as your health status evolves or as you identify new triggers and sensitivities. Maintain flexibility in your environmental setup and be prepared to modify protocols based on changing needs or new information about your specific sensitivities.

The Reality of Environmental Sensitivity

Creating an optimal sleep environment for patients with EDS, POTS, and MCAS isn't about being high-maintenance or overly particular — it's about acknowledging the reality of heightened sensitivities and environmental reactivity that are part of these conditions. Your nervous system and immune system are already stressed by chronic illness; eliminating unnecessary environmental stressors can significantly improve your overall symptom management and sleep quality.

The process of environmental optimization takes time, experimentation, and often significant investment. However, most patients find that systematic attention to environmental factors provides substantial improvements in sleep quality that justify the effort and expense involved.

Family members and partners may initially be skeptical about the need for extensive environmental modifications. Education about the physiological basis for environmental sensitivities and the demonstrated impact on sleep quality can help gain necessary cooperation for maintaining an optimal sleep environment.

Environmental Optimization Success Strategies

The most successful patients approach environmental optimization systematically rather than randomly trying different products or modifications. They document their current environment, prioritize changes based on likely impact and cost-effectiveness, implement modifications gradually to assess individual effects, and maintain their optimized environment through regular monitoring and maintenance.

Remember that your optimal sleep environment may be different from recommendations for other patients with the same conditions. Individual sensitivities and preferences vary significantly, and what works well for one person may be problematic for another. The goal is finding environmental conditions that support your specific needs rather than following generic recommendations.

Environmental optimization is an ongoing process rather than a one-time setup. Your needs may change as your health status evolves, new environmental triggers are identified, or seasonal factors change. Maintaining an optimal sleep environment requires ongoing attention and willingness to make adjustments as needed.

The investment in environmental optimization typically pays dividends in improved sleep quality, reduced symptom severity, and better overall quality of life. For patients whose sleep is significantly impacted by environmental factors, systematic environmental management often provides more benefit than adding medications or other interventions.

Environmental Excellence Fundamentals:

- Implement systematic environmental assessment and modification protocols rather than making random changes
- Address temperature, humidity, air quality, light management, sound control, and chemical elimination in a coordinated approach
- Prioritize cost-effective modifications that address your most significant environmental triggers first

- Maintain your optimized environment through regular cleaning, filter replacement, and equipment maintenance schedules
- Monitor environmental conditions objectively using appropriate measuring devices when possible
- Remain flexible and willing to adjust environmental protocols as your needs change or new sensitivities develop

Chapter 8: Revolutionary Sleep Positioning for Hypermobility

Joint instability during sleep isn't just uncomfortable — it's a systematic assault on your body's attempt to achieve restorative rest. Your joints are supposed to maintain stable positions during sleep, allowing muscles to relax and tissues to repair. But when you have EDS, your joints seem to have their own agenda, subluxating and shifting in ways that jolt you awake just as you're achieving deeper sleep stages. This isn't a minor inconvenience; it's a fundamental disruption of sleep architecture that requires sophisticated positioning strategies.

Most sleep positioning advice assumes you have normal joint stability and average proprioception. That advice is not only useless for hypermobile patients — it can actually make things worse by encouraging positions that stress unstable joints. You need positioning strategies based on understanding joint mechanics, proprioceptive deficits, and the specific vulnerability patterns that occur during different sleep stages.

Position-Specific Protocols

Side Sleeping Optimization for the Majority

Research indicates that 50.7% of patients with hypermobility prefer side sleeping, making this the most common sleep position that needs optimization (The Fibro Guy, 2024). However, side sleeping presents unique challenges for joint stability, particularly for the shoulder, hip, and spine alignment that require specific support strategies.

Shoulder Protection Protocols: The dependent shoulder (the one you're lying on) is at highest risk for anterior subluxation during side sleeping. The weight of your body combined with the pulling force of gravity on your upper arm creates stress that normal joint capsules can resist but hypermobile joints cannot. The solution isn't avoiding side sleeping — it's supporting the shoulder properly.

Position your bottom arm slightly forward of your body rather than directly underneath you. This reduces the compression force on the shoulder joint while maintaining comfortable positioning. Use a contoured pillow designed specifically for side sleepers that has a cutout for the shoulder, reducing pressure while maintaining support for your head and neck.

The top shoulder requires different support to prevent posterior subluxation from the arm falling backward during sleep. Place a pillow or bolster behind your back to prevent rolling too far forward, and use a pillow between your arms to support the top shoulder in a neutral position.

Hip and Pelvis Stabilization: Side sleeping without proper support often leads to hip adduction and internal rotation that can stress the hip joint and sacroiliac joints. The key is maintaining neutral hip alignment throughout the night, even as you move and change positions.

Place a firm pillow between your knees that extends from your thighs to your ankles. This pillow should be thick enough to keep your hips in neutral alignment — typically 4-6 inches for most people, but this varies based on your body proportions and hip width. The pillow should be long enough to support your entire leg, preventing your ankles from rotating inward.

For patients with severe hip instability, consider a full-length body pillow that provides support from your chest to your ankles. This creates a more stable surface that reduces position changes during sleep while maintaining proper joint alignment.

Spinal Alignment Maintenance: Side sleeping can create lateral spinal curves that stress hypermobile joints and compress nerve roots. Your pillow height needs to fill the space between your shoulder and your head while keeping your neck in neutral alignment with your spine.

The correct pillow height depends on your shoulder width and preferred firmness. As a general rule, people with broader shoulders need higher pillows, while those with narrower shoulders need lower support. However, hypermobile patients often need slightly more support than their body proportions would suggest because their joints require more external stabilization.

The Position-Changing Strategy for Restless Sleepers

Research shows that 21.7% of hypermobile patients use frequent position changes as a sleep strategy (The Fibro Guy, 2024). While this might seem disruptive, it can actually be protective if done correctly. The key is facilitating smooth position changes that don't create joint stress while maintaining support throughout the transition.

Transition Support Systems: Create a sleep environment that supports smooth position changes rather than fighting against them. Use multiple pillows of different sizes and firmness levels positioned around your bed so you can easily access support regardless of your position.

Bilateral Positioning Setups: Set up your bed so that you can sleep comfortably on either side without having to rearrange pillows. This means having appropriate pillows on both sides of your bed and ensuring that your mattress provides consistent support regardless of which side you prefer at any given time.

Movement-Friendly Bedding: Choose sheets and blankets that move with you rather than restricting position changes. Fitted sheets should have deep pockets and elastic that maintains position even with movement. Avoid tightly tucked bedding that might restrict movement or create pressure points when you change position.

Monitoring Position Change Patterns: Keep track of how often you change positions and whether certain positions lead to more stable sleep. Some patients find that they need to change positions every 1-2 hours to prevent joint stiffness, while others can maintain one position for longer periods with proper support.

Back Sleeping Modifications for the Few

Only 10.1% of hypermobile patients prefer back sleeping, often because this position can worsen both joint instability and autonomic symptoms (The Fibro Guy, 2024). However, for patients who can tolerate back sleeping, proper modifications can make this a very stable and supportive position.

Cervical Spine Support: Back sleeping requires careful attention to cervical spine positioning because the loss of the natural cervical curve can stress hypermobile neck joints. Use a pillow that maintains the natural cervical curve while supporting the head appropriately.

Many patients benefit from cervical support pillows that have a built-in curve or from placing a small rolled towel under the neck with a flatter pillow supporting the head. The goal is maintaining the natural lordotic curve of the cervical spine while preventing hyperextension or excessive flexion.

Lumbar Support Integration: The lumbar spine often flattens during back sleeping, which can stress hypermobile lumbar joints and create morning stiffness. Place a small pillow or lumbar roll under your knees to flex your hips slightly, which helps maintain the natural lumbar curve.

Some patients benefit from a thin lumbar support pillow placed under the small of their back, but this should be used cautiously because too much lumbar support can actually increase joint stress in some hypermobile patients.

Extremity Positioning: Support your arms and legs to prevent them from falling into positions that might stress joints. Place small pillows under your arms to prevent shoulder internal rotation, and consider a pillow under your ankles to prevent foot drop and maintain neutral ankle positioning.

Why Stomach Sleeping Increases Subluxation Risk

Stomach sleeping forces the cervical spine into rotation and extension that exceeds safe ranges for hypermobile joints. This position also requires significant lumbar extension and often leads to shoulder positioning that stresses the glenohumeral joint capsule.

Cervical Spine Stress Mechanisms: Stomach sleeping requires turning your head to one side for breathing, creating sustained cervical rotation combined with extension. This position stretches the joint capsules and ligaments on one side while compressing structures on the other side. For hypermobile patients, this sustained stress often leads to subluxation or significant stiffness upon waking.

Shoulder Impingement Risks: The arm positioning required for stomach sleeping often places the shoulder in positions that compress soft tissues and stress the joint capsule. The combination of shoulder abduction, external rotation, and elevation can create impingement that develops into pain and instability over time.

Respiratory Compromise: Stomach sleeping can also compromise breathing by restricting chest expansion and potentially triggering POTS symptoms related to reduced oxygen saturation. For patients who absolutely cannot sleep in other positions, modifications include using very thin pillows and ensuring that chest expansion isn't restricted by mattress firmness.

Pillow Engineering Systems

Strategic Five-Pillow Configuration

Effective positioning for hypermobile patients often requires multiple pillows strategically placed to provide support for different body parts simultaneously. This isn't about luxury or comfort — it's about creating external stability for joints that lack internal stability.

Primary Support Pillow (Head and Neck): Choose a pillow that matches your sleeping position and maintains proper cervical alignment. This pillow should be replaced regularly because loss of shape and support can gradually worsen joint positioning without obvious symptoms until significant problems develop.

Knee/Leg Support Pillow: For side sleepers, this pillow maintains hip alignment and prevents internal rotation. For back sleepers, it helps maintain lumbar curve and reduces hip flexor tightness. The pillow should be firm enough to maintain position throughout the night but soft enough to be comfortable for extended contact.

Arm Support Pillow: Provides support for the top arm during side sleeping or for both arms during back sleeping. This pillow prevents shoulder internal rotation and reduces stress on the glenohumeral joint capsule.

Back Support Pillow: For side sleepers, this pillow prevents rolling too far forward and maintains spinal alignment. It should be positioned along your back from your shoulders to your hips to provide consistent support.

Ankle/Foot Support Pillow: Supports the ankles and prevents foot drop, particularly important for patients with ankle instability or peripheral neuropathy. This pillow also helps maintain leg alignment and prevents the bottom leg from rotating inward during side sleeping.

Memory Foam vs. Water vs. Down Alternatives

Different pillow materials provide different types of support that may be more or less appropriate for specific joint stability needs and comfort preferences.

Memory Foam Characteristics: Memory foam provides consistent support that conforms to body contours while maintaining its shape. This can be excellent for joint stability because it provides sustained support without pressure points. However, memory foam can retain heat and may make position changes more difficult because of its slow response to movement.

Temperature-Sensitive Considerations: Traditional memory foam becomes firmer in cold temperatures and softer in warm temperatures. For patients with temperature regulation problems, this variability can be problematic. Gel-infused or plant-based memory foams often provide more temperature stability.

Water Pillow Benefits: Water pillows allow precise adjustment of support level by adding or removing water. This adjustability can be excellent for patients whose support needs change based on symptom severity or for those who need different support levels on different sides of their body.

Maintenance Requirements: Water pillows require more maintenance than other options and can develop leaks over time. However, the precise adjustability often makes this additional maintenance worthwhile for patients with specific support needs.

Down Alternative Advantages: High-quality down alternative pillows can provide good support while being more responsive to movement than memory foam. They're also hypoallergenic and easier to wash than natural down. However, they may require more frequent replacement as they lose loft over time.

Support Longevity: Down alternative pillows often lose support gradually, making it difficult to notice when replacement is needed. Establish a regular replacement schedule rather than waiting for obvious deterioration.

Proprioceptive Feedback Enhancement

Patients with EDS often have impaired proprioception — the ability to sense joint position and movement. Strategic pillow placement can provide enhanced sensory feedback that helps your brain maintain awareness of joint position during sleep.

Contact Surface Optimization: Pillows that provide gentle contact with skin surfaces can enhance proprioceptive feedback without creating pressure points. This contact helps your nervous system maintain awareness of body position even during sleep when conscious awareness is reduced.

Texture Considerations: Some patients benefit from pillows with different textures that provide additional sensory input. However, textures should be subtle enough not to cause irritation during extended contact.

Weight and Pressure Distribution: Weighted elements in pillows can provide proprioceptive feedback through deep pressure stimulation. However, weight should be distributed evenly to avoid creating pressure points or restricting circulation.

Custom Positioning for Individual Subluxation Patterns

Every patient has specific joints that are more prone to subluxation and specific movements or positions that trigger instability. Effective positioning strategies must be customized to address individual vulnerability patterns rather than using generic recommendations.

Joint-Specific Assessments: Identify which joints are most problematic during sleep and what positions or movements tend to trigger symptoms. This assessment should include morning joint status as well as nighttime awakenings related to joint instability.

Pattern Recognition: Track relationships between sleep positioning and morning joint status. Some positions that feel comfortable initially may lead to morning stiffness or instability, while other positions that feel awkward initially may result in better morning joint function.

Adaptive Positioning Strategies: Develop positioning strategies that can be adjusted based on current symptom severity or joint stability. On days when joints are particularly unstable, you may need additional support or different positioning than on days when symptoms are better controlled.

Progressive Positioning Changes: Some patients need to gradually transition to optimal positioning over several weeks because their bodies are accustomed to poor positioning patterns. Sudden changes to optimal positioning can sometimes create discomfort until tissues adapt to better alignment.

Real-World Implementation Challenges

The biggest challenge with sleep positioning for hypermobile patients is that optimal positioning often feels awkward or uncomfortable initially. Your body has adapted to poor positioning patterns, and correcting these patterns requires patience and persistence while your tissues adjust to better alignment.

Partner accommodation can also be challenging when optimal positioning requires multiple pillows or specific bed arrangements. Open communication about the medical necessity of positioning supports can help partners understand that these aren't arbitrary preferences but necessary medical interventions.

The cost of multiple specialized pillows can be significant, but this investment often pays dividends in improved sleep quality and reduced morning pain and stiffness. Consider purchasing pillows gradually, starting with the most important supports and adding additional elements as budget allows.

Maintenance of multiple pillows requires regular washing and replacement schedules. Develop systems for maintaining pillows in good condition and replace them before support deterioration affects joint stability.

Positioning Protocol Success Strategies

Start with basic positioning improvements before investing in expensive specialized equipment. Simple modifications like proper pillow placement often provide significant benefits before more sophisticated interventions are needed.

Document your positioning strategies and their effects on sleep quality and morning joint status. This documentation helps identify which modifications provide the most benefit and guides future positioning optimization.

Be patient with the adaptation process. Optimal positioning may feel uncomfortable initially, but most patients adapt within 2-4 weeks and then find that poor positioning becomes obviously uncomfortable.

Consider working with a physical therapist familiar with hypermobility to develop personalized positioning strategies. Professional guidance can help identify positioning modifications that you might not discover through trial and error alone.

Positioning Excellence Points:

- Implement position-specific support strategies that address the unique joint stability challenges of side sleeping, back sleeping, and position changing
- Use systematic pillow engineering with multiple pillows strategically placed to provide external stability for hypermobile joints
- Choose pillow materials based on support requirements, temperature considerations, and individual comfort preferences
- Customize positioning strategies to address your specific pattern of joint instability and subluxation risks
- Document positioning effectiveness and be patient with the adaptation process while your body adjusts to better alignment
- Consider professional guidance from physical therapists familiar with hypermobility for personalized positioning optimization

Chapter 9: Mattress Selection Science

Your mattress isn't just a place to sleep — it's the foundation that either supports or sabotages every joint stabilization strategy you implement. For patients with hypermobility, the wrong mattress can undo all your careful pillow positioning and environmental optimization within hours. The stakes are higher than comfort; they're about maintaining joint stability throughout the vulnerable hours when your protective muscle tone decreases and your joints become dependent on external support.

The mattress industry loves to make bold claims about "orthopedic support" and "pressure relief," but most of these claims aren't backed by research specific to hypermobile joints. You need a mattress that provides consistent support without creating pressure points, maintains proper spinal alignment during position changes, and responds appropriately to your movement patterns without either trapping you in one position or allowing excessive sinking that destabilizes joints.

Evidence-Based Recommendations

Hybrid Mattresses for Optimal Support

Research consistently demonstrates that hybrid mattresses — combining innerspring coils with memory foam or latex layers — provide the best balance of support and pressure relief for patients with joint instability (Zoma Sleep Research Team, 2024). This combination addresses the dual needs of maintaining spinal alignment while accommodating pressure-sensitive areas around hypermobile joints.

Coil System Requirements: The innerspring component should use individually wrapped coils (pocket coils) rather than interconnected coil systems. Pocket coils respond independently to pressure, providing support where needed while allowing pressure relief in areas that don't require firm support. This independent response is crucial for hypermobile patients whose support needs vary dramatically across different body areas.

The coil gauge (thickness) affects support characteristics significantly. Lower gauge numbers indicate thicker, firmer coils that provide more support but less contouring. For hypermobile patients, 13-15 gauge coils typically provide optimal support without excessive firmness that could create pressure points at bony prominences.

Comfort Layer Integration: The comfort layers above the coils should provide pressure relief without allowing excessive sinking that could destabilize joints. Memory foam layers should be 2-4 inches thick — enough to provide pressure relief but not so thick that you sink deeply enough to compromise spinal alignment.

Latex comfort layers often provide better responsiveness than memory foam, allowing easier position changes while still providing pressure relief. However, latex can be too firm for some pressure-sensitive patients, requiring careful selection based on individual tolerance.

Zoning Technology Benefits: Some hybrid mattresses incorporate zoning technology that provides different firmness levels for different body areas. Firmer zones under the torso maintain spinal alignment, while softer zones under the hips and shoulders provide pressure relief. This technology can be particularly beneficial for hypermobile patients whose support needs vary significantly between body regions.

Memory Foam Benefits and Limitations

Memory foam provides excellent pressure relief and can help reduce joint stress by distributing weight evenly across the sleeping surface. However, traditional memory foam also has characteristics that can be problematic for some hypermobile patients.

Pressure Relief Advantages: Memory foam excels at eliminating pressure points by conforming closely to body contours. For patients with joint pain or pressure sensitivity, this conforming characteristic can provide significant comfort improvements. The material responds to body heat and pressure, creating a custom-fitting surface that adapts to individual body shape.

Temperature Considerations: Traditional memory foam retains body heat, which can be problematic for patients with temperature regulation issues. Gel-infused memory foam, plant-based foams, or open-cell foam constructions provide better temperature regulation while maintaining pressure relief benefits.

Response Time Limitations: Memory foam's slow response to movement can make position changes more difficult and may create a "trapped" feeling that some patients find claustrophobic. This slow response can also mean that support doesn't adjust quickly when you change positions, potentially creating temporary joint stress during transitions.

Density Requirements: Memory foam density affects both support and durability. Higher density foams (4-6 pounds per cubic foot) provide better support and last longer but may feel firmer and retain more heat. Lower density foams are softer and cooler but may not provide adequate support for joint stability and may deteriorate more quickly.

Firmness Selection by Body Type and Joint Patterns

Optimal firmness for hypermobile patients depends on body weight, primary sleep position, and specific pattern of joint instability. The goal is finding firmness that maintains spinal alignment while providing pressure relief for sensitive joints.

Body Weight Considerations: Heavier individuals typically need firmer mattresses to prevent excessive sinking that compromises spinal alignment. However, hypermobile patients may need slightly softer surfaces than their body weight would typically require because they often have increased pressure sensitivity around unstable joints.

Sleep Position Requirements: Side sleepers generally need softer surfaces to accommodate hip and shoulder pressure, while back sleepers need firmer support to maintain spinal alignment. Combination sleepers need surfaces that work reasonably well for multiple positions rather than being optimized for one specific position.

Joint Instability Patterns: Patients with primarily spinal instability may need firmer overall support, while those with peripheral joint problems (shoulders, hips) may prioritize pressure relief in these areas. Some patients need firmer support under the torso with softer areas for pressure-sensitive extremities.

Firmness Scale Understanding: Mattress firmness is typically rated on a 1-10 scale, but these ratings aren't standardized across manufacturers. Most hypermobile patients find optimal comfort in the 5-7 range (medium to medium-firm), but individual preferences can vary significantly based on specific joint problems and pressure sensitivity patterns.

Implementation Protocols

90-120 Day Trial Period Optimization

Most quality mattress manufacturers offer trial periods that allow you to test the mattress at home for extended periods. For hypermobile patients, this trial period is essential because mattress suitability often isn't apparent during brief store testing.

Week 1-2: Initial Adaptation Your body needs time to adapt to new support patterns, and initial discomfort doesn't necessarily indicate that a mattress is inappropriate. Document sleep quality, morning joint status, and any specific comfort issues during this initial period.

Week 3-6: Assessment Period By the third week, adaptation issues should be resolving, and you can begin meaningful assessment of mattress performance. Focus on:

- Morning joint stiffness or pain patterns
- Sleep continuity and awakening frequency
- Pressure point development
- Overall comfort and support satisfaction

- Partner comfort and motion isolation (if applicable)

Week 7-12: Final Evaluation Use this period for fine-tuning with mattress toppers or adjusting your pillow configuration. Some mattresses may require accessories to optimize performance for individual needs.

Documentation Strategies: Keep detailed records of sleep quality, joint symptoms, and overall satisfaction throughout the trial period. This documentation helps with return decisions and provides valuable information for future mattress selection if the current choice doesn't work out.

Assessment Metrics for Success

Successful mattress selection should be measured by objective improvements in sleep quality and joint function rather than just subjective comfort impressions.

Sleep Quality Metrics:

- Reduced frequency of awakening due to joint discomfort
- Decreased time needed to fall asleep
- Improved morning energy levels
- Reduced need for position changes during sleep
- Better overall sleep satisfaction scores

Joint Function Assessment:

- Reduced morning joint stiffness
- Decreased morning pain levels
- Improved joint stability upon waking
- Reduced frequency of nighttime subluxations
- Better overall joint function throughout the day

Pressure Point Evaluation:

- Absence of pressure-related pain upon waking

- No development of pressure sores or skin irritation
- Comfortable weight distribution without pressure concentration
- Appropriate support for pressure-sensitive areas

Partner Considerations: If you share your bed, assess impact on your partner's sleep quality and comfort. Motion isolation, temperature regulation, and edge support may be important factors for partner satisfaction.

When to Upgrade vs. Modify Existing Setup

Not every sleep surface problem requires complete mattress replacement. Sometimes modifications can provide significant improvements at much lower cost and effort.

Mattress Topper Solutions: High-quality mattress toppers can modify the feel and support characteristics of existing mattresses significantly. Memory foam toppers can add pressure relief to firm mattresses, while latex toppers can add responsiveness to memory foam mattresses.

Support Enhancement: If your current mattress is comfortable but lacks adequate support, box spring replacement or foundation upgrades can sometimes provide needed support improvements without requiring complete mattress replacement.

Temperature Regulation Additions: Cooling mattress pads, breathable protectors, or temperature-regulating toppers can address temperature issues without mattress replacement.

When Replacement is Necessary:

- Significant sagging or permanent indentations
- Loss of support that can't be corrected with toppers
- Development of pressure points that can't be relieved with modifications
- Temperature problems that can't be addressed with accessories
- Overall deterioration that affects sleep quality significantly

Insurance and Medical Necessity Documentation

Some health insurance plans or flexible spending accounts may cover mattresses prescribed for medical conditions. Documentation from healthcare providers about the medical necessity of proper sleep support can help with reimbursement efforts.

Medical Documentation Requirements: Obtain documentation from your physician that describes how your specific medical conditions require specialized sleep support. This documentation should reference your diagnosed conditions (EDS, POTS, MCAS) and explain how proper sleep support is medically necessary for managing these conditions.

Prescription Requirements: Some insurance plans require formal prescriptions for durable medical equipment, which may include therapeutic mattresses. Work with your healthcare provider to determine if a formal prescription would be helpful for insurance coverage.

Cost-Benefit Analysis: Document the costs of poor sleep support, including increased medical visits, medication needs, and lost productivity. This information can support arguments for coverage of appropriate sleep support equipment.

Budget-Friendly Alternatives That Work

High-quality sleep support doesn't always require expensive mattresses. Several strategies can provide significant improvements in support and comfort without major financial investment.

Mattress Topper Combinations: Strategic use of multiple mattress toppers can create customized support systems at fraction of the cost of new mattresses. Combining firm support toppers with pressure-relieving comfort layers allows fine-tuning of support characteristics.

DIY Support Modifications: Plywood boards between mattresses and box springs can increase support for sagging mattresses. Strategic pillow placement can provide targeted support for specific body areas without requiring mattress replacement.

Phased Improvement Strategies: Implement improvements gradually as budget allows. Start with essential modifications like supportive pillows and mattress toppers, then progress to more expensive improvements as needed and affordable.

Quality Used Options: Consider certified refurbished mattresses from reputable manufacturers. These options can provide significant cost savings while still offering quality materials and construction.

The Mattress Selection Reality

Choosing the right mattress for hypermobile patients requires balancing multiple factors that often seem contradictory — you need support that prevents joint instability but pressure relief that accommodates sensitive areas. You need responsiveness that allows position changes but stability that prevents excessive movement. These competing needs mean that mattress selection often involves compromise and fine-tuning rather than finding perfect solutions.

The mattress industry's marketing claims often exceed the actual benefits their products provide. Focus on fundamental characteristics like coil quality, foam density, and overall construction rather than proprietary technologies that may not provide meaningful benefits for your specific needs.

Trial periods are essential because mattress suitability for hypermobile patients often isn't apparent during brief testing. Use trial periods systematically to assess objective improvements in sleep quality and joint function rather than just subjective comfort impressions.

Mattress Mastery Strategies:

- Choose hybrid mattresses with individually wrapped coils and appropriate comfort layers for optimal balance of support and pressure relief

- Use extended trial periods systematically to assess objective improvements in sleep quality and joint function
- Consider firmness requirements based on body weight, sleep position, and specific joint instability patterns
- Implement cost-effective modifications with toppers and accessories before investing in complete mattress replacement
- Document medical necessity for insurance coverage consideration and maintain detailed records of mattress performance
- Focus on fundamental mattress characteristics rather than marketing claims when making selection decisions

Chapter 10: Compression and Bracing Strategies

Compression garments and supportive bracing during sleep walk a fine line between providing essential joint stability and creating circulation problems that can worsen your symptoms. For hypermobile patients, the question isn't whether to use compression during sleep — it's how to use it safely and effectively without creating new problems while you address existing joint instability.

The challenge lies in the fact that your circulation changes dramatically during sleep, your position tolerance varies throughout the night, and the compression that feels supportive while awake might become problematic during extended sleep periods. You need strategies that provide stability when needed while accommodating the physiological changes that occur during different sleep stages.

Sleep-Safe Support Systems

Compression Garment Protocols for Extended Use

The compression levels that work well during daytime activities often need modification for nighttime use because circulation changes, position tolerance shifts, and extended contact with skin requires different material considerations. Research indicates that compression levels of 15-30 mmHg provide optimal therapeutic benefit for most hypermobile patients while remaining safe for extended use (Sheldon et al., 2015).

Graduated Compression Principles: Effective compression garments use graduated pressure that's highest at the extremities and decreases toward the core. This pressure gradient helps promote venous return while providing joint support. However, during sleep, position changes can alter the effectiveness of graduated compression, requiring garments designed specifically for extended horizontal positioning.

Material Considerations for Extended Wear: Sleep-appropriate compression garments require materials that maintain compression while allowing moisture wicking and temperature regulation. Look for garments with:

- Breathable synthetic fibers that wick moisture away from skin
- Flat seams that won't create pressure points during extended contact
- Appropriate stretch characteristics that maintain compression without becoming too tight as swelling patterns change during sleep
- Hypoallergenic materials that won't trigger skin reactions during extended contact

Pressure Level Modifications: Daytime compression levels may be too high for safe nighttime use. Consider reducing compression levels by 5-10 mmHg for sleep use, or choose garments specifically designed for nighttime wear that provide adequate support with lower pressure levels.

Application Timing and Technique: Apply compression garments 30-60 minutes before bedtime to allow circulation adjustment before lying down. Ensure proper fit without wrinkles or tight spots that could create pressure points during extended wear. Check circulation in fingers and toes after application to ensure adequate blood flow.

Strategic Bracing for Unstable Joints

Nighttime bracing presents unique challenges because protective devices that work well during waking hours may become uncomfortable or even dangerous during sleep when you can't monitor their effects or adjust positioning as needed.

Joint-Specific Bracing Considerations:

Knee Bracing for Sleep: Knee instability during sleep often involves lateral movement that can stress the joint capsule or create patellar tracking problems. Simple knee sleeves that provide mild compression and proprioceptive feedback are often more appropriate for sleep than rigid braces that might restrict necessary position changes.

For patients with severe knee instability, consider soft hinged braces that allow flexion and extension while limiting lateral movement. These braces should have padding in areas that contact the bed and should be loose enough to accommodate circulation changes during sleep.

Ankle Support Systems: Ankle instability during sleep can lead to inversion injuries or stress on already-compromised ligaments. Soft ankle braces or compression sleeves that provide support without rigidity often work best for sleep use.

Avoid lace-up ankle braces during sleep because the laces can create pressure points or become too tight as foot swelling changes throughout the night. Slip-on designs with adjustable straps or compression sleeves provide support with better tolerance for circulation changes.

Wrist and Hand Bracing: Wrist subluxations during sleep are common, particularly in side sleepers who place weight on their hands or arms. Soft wrist braces that maintain neutral positioning without completely immobilizing the joint provide protection while allowing necessary movement.

For patients with thumb instability, thumb spica splints designed for extended wear can prevent hyperextension injuries during sleep. These should be made from soft materials with adequate padding to prevent pressure sores.

Proprioceptive Feedback Garments

Some patients benefit from garments that provide sensory input to help maintain joint position awareness even during sleep when conscious proprioception is reduced. These garments work by providing gentle contact pressure that enhances the nervous system's ability to track joint position.

Compression Shirts for Torso Stability: Lightweight compression shirts can provide proprioceptive feedback for spinal positioning while offering mild support for shoulder positioning. Choose garments with appropriate compression levels that provide sensory input without restricting breathing or circulation.

Compression Shorts for Hip Stability: Compression shorts can help with hip positioning and provide support for sacroiliac joint stability during sleep. Look for designs that don't create binding in the groin area and that maintain compression without becoming too tight as position changes occur.

Combination Garments: Some manufacturers produce garments that combine compression with targeted support for multiple joints. These can be efficient for patients who need support for several areas but should be evaluated carefully to ensure they don't create pressure points or circulation problems.

Safety Monitoring and Skin Protection

Extended use of compression garments and braces requires vigilant monitoring for circulation problems, pressure sores, and skin irritation that might develop during sleep when you can't consciously assess comfort and safety.

Circulation Monitoring Protocols: Before sleep, check that compression garments aren't too tight by ensuring you can slide one finger under the garment easily. Check fingernails and toenails for color changes that might indicate circulation problems. If you wake during the night, briefly assess sensation and circulation in compressed areas.

Skin Protection Strategies: Use barrier creams or powders in areas prone to moisture accumulation under compression garments. Pay particular attention to skin folds and areas where seams contact skin. Rotate compression garments daily to allow skin recovery and prevent breakdown from constant pressure.

Warning Signs Requiring Immediate Removal:

- Numbness or tingling that doesn't resolve quickly after position changes
- Color changes in extremities (blue, gray, or white coloration)
- Significant swelling above or below compression garments
- Skin breakdown, redness, or irritation that doesn't resolve quickly
- Pain that seems related to compression rather than underlying joint problems

Partner Monitoring: If you sleep with a partner, educate them about signs of circulation problems that might require waking you to remove compression garments. This backup monitoring can be important for safety during deep sleep when you might not notice circulation changes.

Implementation and Adjustment Strategies

Gradual Introduction Protocols

Starting compression and bracing protocols gradually allows your circulation system to adapt while helping you identify optimal garment choices and compression levels for your individual needs.

Week 1-2: Daytime Tolerance Assessment Begin by using compression garments during daytime hours to assess tolerance and identify any skin sensitivity or circulation issues. Start with lower compression levels and gradually increase as tolerated.

Week 3-4: Short Nighttime Trials Begin with 2-4 hour nighttime trials during naps or early evening rest periods. This allows assessment of nighttime tolerance while maintaining the ability to remove garments easily if problems develop.

Week 5-6: Full Night Implementation Progress to full nighttime use only after demonstrating good tolerance during shorter trials. Continue to monitor carefully for the first several weeks of full nighttime use.

Individual Customization Requirements

Effective compression and bracing strategies must be tailored to individual patterns of joint instability, circulation characteristics, and comfort preferences. Generic recommendations often fail because individual variations in anatomy, symptom patterns, and tolerance levels are significant.

Joint Priority Assessment: Identify which joints are most problematic during sleep and prioritize support for these areas. Don't try to support every potentially unstable joint simultaneously — focus on the most problematic areas first and add additional support gradually as needed and tolerated.

Circulation Pattern Evaluation: Assess your individual circulation patterns and how they change during sleep. Some patients develop more swelling in extremities during sleep, while others experience circulation improvement in horizontal positions. Tailor compression strategies to your individual circulation characteristics.

Comfort and Tolerance Factors: Consider individual factors like skin sensitivity, temperature tolerance, and claustrophobia that might affect garment selection. Some patients tolerate firm compression well, while others need very light pressure to avoid triggering anxiety or circulation problems.

The Practical Reality of Sleep Compression

The biggest challenge with compression and bracing during sleep is balancing the need for joint support with the risks of circulation compromise and comfort problems during extended use. This balance is different for every patient and may change as your condition evolves or as your tolerance for compression changes.

Many patients find that the compression garments they use successfully during the day are too restrictive or uncomfortable for nighttime use. This often requires purchasing separate garments designed specifically for sleep use, which can be expensive but is often necessary for safe and effective nighttime support.

Partner accommodation can be challenging when compression garments or braces affect comfort during shared sleep space. Open communication about the medical necessity of these interventions helps partners understand that these aren't optional preferences but necessary medical treatments.

The psychological aspect of using compression garments during sleep shouldn't be underestimated. Some patients find compression comforting and stabilizing, while others experience anxiety or claustrophobia. Individual tolerance for compression often influences success more than the theoretical benefits of specific garment designs.

Strategic Support Implementation

Success with compression and bracing during sleep requires systematic approach that prioritizes safety while maximizing therapeutic benefit. Start with the most problematic joints and use the minimum compression needed to provide benefit. Monitor carefully for circulation problems and skin issues that might develop with extended use.

Document your experiences with different garment types, compression levels, and application techniques. This documentation helps optimize your compression strategy and provides valuable information for healthcare providers who might need to recommend specific products or techniques.

Be prepared to modify your compression strategy based on changes in your condition, seasonal factors, or activity levels that might affect your tolerance for compression. Flexibility in approach often leads to better long-term success than rigid adherence to specific protocols.

Consider working with occupational therapists or orthotists who have experience with hypermobility and compression garment prescription.

Professional guidance can help you avoid common mistakes and identify appropriate products for your specific needs.

Compression and Bracing Excellence Guidelines:

- Use sleep-appropriate compression levels (15-30 mmHg) with materials designed for extended wear and moisture management
- Implement gradual introduction protocols to assess tolerance and identify optimal garment choices
- Prioritize safety monitoring for circulation problems and skin protection during extended use
- Customize compression strategies to individual joint instability patterns and comfort tolerance
- Document garment performance and work with healthcare professionals familiar with hypermobility
- Maintain flexibility to modify compression strategies based on changing needs and tolerance

Key Implementation Strategies:

- Begin with lower compression levels and gradually increase as tolerance develops
- Choose garments specifically designed for extended wear rather than modifying daytime compression
- Monitor circulation and skin condition vigilantly during initial implementation periods
- Prioritize joint support based on individual instability patterns rather than trying to support everything simultaneously
- Maintain backup monitoring through educated partners for safety during deep sleep periods
- Work with healthcare professionals to ensure appropriate garment selection and safe implementation protocols

Chapter 11: Mast Cell Stabilization Mastery

The pharmaceutical management of mast cell activation doesn't follow the neat patterns that drug companies would like you to believe. Your mast cells aren't reading the prescribing information, and they certainly don't care about standard dosing recommendations that were developed for people without hyperreactive immune systems. Getting effective mast cell stabilization requires understanding both the science behind these medications and the practical realities of implementing them in bodies that react unpredictably to pharmaceutical interventions.

The biggest mistake patients make is expecting immediate results from mast cell stabilizers. These medications work by preventing degranulation rather than treating symptoms after they occur, which means you need sustained blood levels and consistent tissue penetration to see benefits. This process takes weeks to months, not hours or days, and requires patience that's hard to maintain when you're suffering from daily symptoms.

Pharmaceutical Protocols

H1/H2 Blocker Timing for 24-Hour Coverage

Antihistamines aren't just for treating allergic reactions — they're the foundation of mast cell management that needs to provide round-the-clock protection against histamine surges. The challenge lies in timing different classes of antihistamines to provide overlapping coverage while avoiding excessive sedation or other side effects.

H1 Antihistamine Scheduling: First-generation H1 antihistamines like diphenhydramine have short half-lives (4-6 hours) but provide potent symptom relief. Second-generation antihistamines like cetirizine or loratadine have longer half-lives (12-24 hours) but may be less effective for severe breakthrough symptoms. The most effective approach often combines both types with strategic timing.

Take your long-acting H1 antihistamine at the same time each day to maintain baseline coverage. Many patients find that morning dosing works well because these medications can provide energy-boosting effects in addition to antihistamine activity. For the 2-4am histamine surge protection, add a short-acting H1 antihistamine around 11pm-midnight to provide peak coverage during vulnerable hours.

H2 Antihistamine Integration: H2 antihistamines like famotidine work on different histamine receptors and provide complementary protection. These medications also help with gastric acid control, which can be beneficial since many MCAS patients have gastrointestinal symptoms. Take H2 antihistamines twice daily — morning and evening — to provide consistent coverage.

Combination Strategies for Severe Cases: Some patients require multiple H1 antihistamines simultaneously to achieve adequate symptom control. This approach should be done under medical supervision, but research supports using up to four different antihistamines daily for severe mast cell disorders (Afrin & Molderings, 2017). The key is avoiding excessive sedation while maximizing histamine receptor blockade.

Timing Optimization:

- **Morning (7-8am):** Long-acting H1 antihistamine + H2 antihistamine
- **Afternoon (2-3pm):** Additional H1 if breakthrough symptoms occur
- **Evening (6-7pm):** Second H2 antihistamine dose
- **Bedtime (10-11pm):** Short-acting H1 for overnight protection

Mast Cell Stabilizer Implementation Timeline

True mast cell stabilizers work differently from antihistamines — they prevent degranulation rather than blocking the effects of released mediators. This difference in mechanism means they require different dosing strategies and patience for effectiveness to develop.

Quercetin Implementation: Start quercetin at 250mg twice daily with meals to assess tolerance. Many patients experience mild gastrointestinal upset initially, which usually resolves within 1-2 weeks. Increase gradually to 500mg twice daily, then to 500mg three times daily if needed for symptom control.

Take quercetin with bromelain and vitamin C to enhance absorption and effectiveness. The combination works synergistically — bromelain helps with quercetin absorption while vitamin C provides additional mast cell stabilizing effects. Expect 4-6 weeks of consistent use before seeing significant symptom improvement.

Cromolyn Sodium Protocols: Prescription cromolyn sodium (gastrocrom) is one of the most effective mast cell stabilizers available, but it requires careful timing and preparation. Take cromolyn 30 minutes before meals on an empty stomach for optimal absorption. The standard dose is 200mg four times daily, but some patients need higher doses under medical supervision.

Cromolyn often causes initial worsening of symptoms (a "herxheimer-like" reaction) as degranulation patterns change. This temporary worsening usually lasts 1-2 weeks and indicates that the medication is working. Don't discontinue during this period unless symptoms become severe.

Ketotifen as Dual-Action Sleep Aid: Ketotifen combines mast cell stabilization with H1 antihistamine activity, making it particularly useful for nighttime dosing. The typical dose is 1mg twice daily, with the evening dose timed 2-3 hours before bedtime to provide sedation for sleep onset while stabilizing mast cells during vulnerable overnight hours.

Start ketotifen at 0.5mg daily and increase gradually because initial sedation can be overwhelming. The sedating effects usually decrease over 2-3 weeks as tolerance develops, but the mast cell stabilizing effects continue. Some patients find that taking the full daily dose at bedtime provides better sleep benefits than divided dosing.

Managing the 12-Month Therapeutic Window

Mast cell stabilizers often show their greatest effectiveness after 6-12 months of consistent use, but many patients discontinue treatment during the first few months due to side effects or perceived lack of effectiveness. Understanding this therapeutic timeline helps maintain treatment adherence during challenging initial periods.

Months 1-3: Foundation Building Focus on establishing tolerance and consistent dosing during this period. Side effects are most common during these initial months, but they usually resolve with continued use. Document symptoms carefully to track subtle improvements that might not be immediately obvious.

Months 4-6: Early Benefits Most patients begin noticing symptom improvements during this period, particularly in sleep quality and digestive symptoms. Energy levels often improve before other symptoms, providing motivation to continue treatment.

Months 7-12: Optimal Effectiveness Maximum benefits typically occur during this period, with continued improvement in symptom severity and frequency. Some patients experience dramatic improvements that weren't apparent during earlier months.

Long-term Maintenance: After achieving optimal benefits, many patients can reduce doses while maintaining symptom control. However, discontinuation often leads to symptom return within weeks to months, indicating the need for long-term treatment in most cases.

Natural Stabilization Strategies

Quercetin Protocols for Maximum Effectiveness

Quercetin is one of the most effective natural mast cell stabilizers, but its benefits depend heavily on proper dosing, timing, and combination with other nutrients that enhance its absorption and effectiveness.

Dosing Strategies: The effective dose range for mast cell stabilization is 500-1000mg daily, divided into 2-3 doses. Lower doses may provide antioxidant benefits but insufficient mast cell stabilization. Higher doses (above 1000mg daily) may cause gastrointestinal upset without additional benefits.

Absorption Enhancement: Quercetin has poor bioavailability when taken alone. Combine with bromelain (100-200mg) to improve absorption, and take with vitamin C (500-1000mg) for synergistic mast cell stabilizing effects. Taking quercetin with a small amount of fat (like nuts or olive oil) also improves absorption.

Timing Optimization: Take quercetin 30 minutes before meals for best absorption. For sleep benefits, take the largest dose 2-3 hours before bedtime to allow time for absorption and tissue distribution. Divide daily doses to maintain consistent blood levels throughout the day.

Quality Considerations: Choose quercetin supplements that specify the form (quercetin dihydrate is most common) and third-party testing for purity. Some forms like quercetin phytosome or liposomal quercetin may have better absorption but are significantly more expensive.

Luteolin and Curcumin Integration

These natural compounds work through different pathways than quercetin, allowing for synergistic benefits when used in combination. Both have anti-inflammatory effects that complement their mast cell stabilizing properties.

Luteolin Implementation: Luteolin is particularly effective for neuroinflammation and may help with the cognitive symptoms (brain fog) common in MCAS patients. The effective dose is 100-200mg daily, taken with meals to reduce gastrointestinal irritation.

Luteolin sources include supplements derived from artichoke leaf extract or synthetic forms. Natural sources tend to be better tolerated but may have variable potency. Start with lower doses because luteolin can cause drowsiness in some patients.

Curcumin Optimization: Curcumin requires enhancement for absorption because it's poorly bioavailable alone. Look for forms combined with piperine (black pepper extract) or phosphatidylserine, or choose liposomal curcumin formulations.

The effective dose for anti-inflammatory effects is 500-1000mg daily of enhanced curcumin. Take with meals containing fat for optimal absorption. Curcumin can interact with certain medications, particularly blood thinners, so medical supervision may be needed.

Combination Protocols: Use quercetin as the foundation mast cell stabilizer, add luteolin for neuroinflammation, and include curcumin for systemic anti-inflammatory effects. This combination provides broader coverage than any single compound alone.

Magnesium Forms and Timing for Nervous System Support

Magnesium deficiency is common in MCAS patients and can worsen mast cell reactivity. Different forms of magnesium have different therapeutic targets, allowing for customized supplementation based on individual symptoms.

Magnesium Glycinate for Sleep: This form is well-absorbed and has calming effects on the nervous system. Take 200-400mg of magnesium glycinate 1-2 hours before bedtime for sleep support and overnight mast cell stabilization.

Magnesium Taurate for Cardiovascular Support: Patients with POTS often benefit from magnesium taurate, which supports cardiovascular function in addition to mast cell stabilization. Take 200-400mg daily, divided between morning and evening doses.

Magnesium Malate for Energy: This form may help with energy production and muscle function. Take 200-400mg with breakfast to support daytime energy levels without interfering with sleep.

Dosing and Timing Strategies: Start with 200mg daily and increase gradually to assess tolerance. Magnesium can cause loose stools if doses are too high or increased too quickly. Space doses throughout the day for better absorption and tolerance.

Synergistic Supplement Combinations

Effective natural mast cell stabilization often requires combinations of supplements that work through different mechanisms. The goal is creating comprehensive mast cell stabilization while avoiding excessive supplement burden.

Foundation Protocol:

- Quercetin 500mg twice daily with bromelain and vitamin C
- Magnesium glycinate 200mg twice daily
- Vitamin D3 2000-4000 IU daily (maintain blood levels 50-80 ng/mL)
- Omega-3 fatty acids 1000-2000mg daily for anti-inflammatory effects

Enhanced Protocol for Severe Symptoms:

- Foundation protocol plus:
- Luteolin 100mg daily
- Curcumin 500mg daily (enhanced absorption form)
- N-acetylcysteine 600mg twice daily for glutathione support
- Vitamin B6 50mg daily to support histamine metabolism

Timing Strategy:

- Morning: Vitamin D3, omega-3, first doses of quercetin and magnesium
- Afternoon: Curcumin, NAC, vitamin B6
- Evening: Second doses of quercetin and magnesium, luteolin

Implementation Challenges and Solutions

Managing Initial Symptom Worsening

Many mast cell stabilizers cause temporary symptom worsening during the first 1-3 weeks of treatment. This occurs because stabilizers change degranulation patterns, often causing initial increased release before achieving stabilization.

Distinguishing Treatment Effects from Disease Progression: Initial worsening from mast cell stabilizers typically involves increased fatigue, mild digestive upset, or temporary increase in usual symptoms. True allergic reactions involve new symptoms like rash, breathing difficulty, or severe reactions not typical of your usual pattern.

Support Strategies During Initial Period:

- Increase antihistamine doses temporarily during initial weeks
- Start new stabilizers one at a time to identify problematic agents
- Use extra environmental precautions to avoid triggers during vulnerable period
- Maintain detailed symptom logs to track patterns versus random fluctuations

Cost-Effectiveness Strategies

Mast cell stabilization can become expensive, particularly when using multiple supplements or prescription medications. Prioritizing interventions based on effectiveness and cost helps maintain treatment adherence.

Priority Ranking:

1. H1 and H2 antihistamines (generic versions are cost-effective)
2. Quercetin with absorption enhancers (good effectiveness-to-cost ratio)
3. Magnesium supplementation (inexpensive with broad benefits)

4. Prescription mast cell stabilizers if natural approaches insufficient
5. Additional natural compounds based on individual response

Money-Saving Approaches:

- Buy supplements in bulk when possible
- Choose generic antihistamines over brand names
- Start with single agents before adding combinations
- Use patient assistance programs for expensive prescription medications
- Consider compounding pharmacies for custom formulations

Long-Term Success Strategies

Monitoring and Adjustment Protocols

Effective mast cell stabilization requires ongoing monitoring and periodic adjustments based on symptom patterns, trigger exposures, and life changes that might affect treatment needs.

Symptom Tracking Systems: Maintain detailed logs of symptoms, triggers, and treatment responses. Look for patterns in symptom severity, timing, and relationship to treatment changes. Use rating scales (1-10) for consistency in tracking improvements or setbacks.

Treatment Response Assessment: Evaluate treatment effectiveness every 3-6 months using objective measures like sleep quality, energy levels, digestive symptoms, and reaction frequency. Adjust doses or agents based on response patterns rather than arbitrary timelines.

Seasonal and Life Stage Adjustments: Many patients need treatment adjustments based on seasonal allergen exposure, hormonal changes, stress levels, or other life factors. Build flexibility into treatment protocols to accommodate these variations.

Integration with Medical Care

Natural mast cell stabilization can complement but shouldn't replace appropriate medical care for severe symptoms. Work with healthcare providers who understand mast cell disorders and are open to integrative approaches.

Communication Strategies:

- Bring research supporting natural approaches to medical appointments
- Document treatment responses objectively to demonstrate effectiveness
- Be open about all supplements and medications you're using
- Seek providers familiar with mast cell disorders when possible

Safety Monitoring: Some natural supplements can interact with medications or have contraindications in certain medical conditions. Regular monitoring may be needed for liver function, blood counts, or other parameters depending on your specific treatment protocol.

The Stabilization Success Framework

Successful mast cell stabilization requires patience, persistence, and willingness to adjust approaches based on individual response patterns. The framework that works best involves:

1. **Foundation establishment** with antihistamines and basic natural stabilizers
2. **Gradual progression** adding agents slowly to assess individual contributions
3. **Consistent implementation** for sufficient time to achieve benefits
4. **Ongoing monitoring** and adjustment based on response patterns
5. **Integration with lifestyle** modifications that support overall mast cell stability

The goal isn't eliminating all mast cell activity — it's achieving stable, appropriate responses that don't interfere with daily functioning and sleep quality. Most patients achieve significant improvement with consistent application of these principles, though individual responses vary considerably.

Stabilization Mastery Framework:

- Implement strategic timing of H1/H2 antihistamines to provide 24-hour coverage with peak protection during vulnerable periods
- Use mast cell stabilizers consistently for 6-12 months to achieve optimal therapeutic benefits
- Combine natural stabilizers synergistically with proper dosing, timing, and absorption enhancement
- Expect initial symptom worsening with stabilizers and plan support strategies for this adjustment period
- Monitor treatment responses objectively and adjust protocols based on individual patterns rather than generic recommendations
- Work with healthcare providers familiar with mast cell disorders while maintaining safety monitoring for supplement interactions

Chapter 12: Autonomic Dysfunction Management at Night

Your autonomic nervous system during sleep is supposed to shift into parasympathetic dominance — the "rest and digest" mode that allows restorative processes to occur. But in POTS patients, this normal shift often fails completely, leaving you in a state of sympathetic hyperarousal that makes sleep onset nearly impossible and sleep maintenance extremely fragmented. This isn't just annoying; it's physiologically disruptive to every system in your body that depends on parasympathetic recovery periods.

The "wired but tired" phenomenon isn't psychological or motivational — it's documented autonomic dysfunction that requires targeted interventions. Your heart rate variability studies probably show reduced parasympathetic activity and excessive sympathetic predominance, particularly during evening hours when your nervous system should be winding down for sleep. Understanding these patterns allows for strategic interventions that can restore more normal autonomic balance during sleep hours.

"Wired but Tired" Solutions

Beta-Blocker Timing and Dosing for Sleep

Beta-blockers can be tremendously helpful for managing the cardiovascular symptoms of POTS, but their timing and dosing for sleep optimization requires careful consideration. The goal is reducing sympathetic hyperarousal without creating excessive hypotension that might worsen orthostatic symptoms in the morning.

Short-Acting vs. Long-Acting Considerations: Propranolol (short-acting) allows more precise timing for evening symptoms but requires multiple daily doses. Metoprolol or atenolol (longer-acting) provide more consistent coverage but may cause morning fatigue if doses are too high. Many patients find that a combination approach works best

— long-acting beta-blockers for baseline coverage with short-acting doses for specific symptom management.

Evening Dosing Strategies: Take evening beta-blocker doses 2-3 hours before bedtime to allow peak effect during sleep onset. This timing provides maximum heart rate control during the vulnerable period when sympathetic hyperarousal typically prevents sleep, while allowing some medication clearance before morning orthostatic challenges.

Sleep-Specific Dosing: Evening beta-blocker doses often need to be higher than morning doses because sympathetic activity typically peaks in the evening hours in POTS patients. Work with your cardiologist to develop different dosing strategies for different times of day based on your individual symptom patterns.

Monitoring and Safety: Check heart rate and blood pressure regularly when adjusting beta-blocker timing or doses. Some patients experience excessive bradycardia (slow heart rate) or hypotension with evening dosing that can be dangerous. Use home monitoring equipment to track responses and adjust doses accordingly.

Central Sympatholytic Strategies

Medications that work in the brain to reduce sympathetic outflow can be particularly effective for the "wired but tired" phenomenon because they address the central nervous system dysfunction rather than just peripheral symptoms.

Clonidine for Sleep Onset: Low-dose clonidine (0.1-0.2mg) taken 1-2 hours before bedtime can help reduce central sympathetic activity and promote sleep onset. This medication works by activating alpha-2 adrenergic receptors in the brain that reduce sympathetic outflow.

Clonidine can cause significant hypotension, particularly in the morning, so blood pressure monitoring is essential. Start with very low doses (0.05mg) and increase gradually based on effectiveness and tolerance. Some patients find that clonidine patches provide more consistent effects with fewer side effects than oral dosing.

Guanfacine as Alternative: Guanfacine works similarly to clonidine but has a longer half-life and may cause less rebound hypertension if missed doses occur. The typical dose for sleep support is 0.5-1mg taken before bedtime.

Methyldopa for Resistant Cases: For patients who don't respond to other central sympatholytics, methyldopa can provide effective sympathetic reduction. However, this medication can cause significant sedation and depression in some patients, requiring careful monitoring.

Vagal Tone Improvement Techniques

The vagus nerve is the primary parasympathetic nerve, and improving vagal tone can help shift autonomic balance toward the parasympathetic dominance needed for restorative sleep. These techniques can be particularly effective when combined with appropriate medications.

Controlled Breathing Exercises: Slow, controlled breathing activates the parasympathetic nervous system through vagal stimulation. The most effective technique is 4-7-8 breathing: inhale for 4 counts, hold for 7 counts, exhale for 8 counts. Practice this technique for 10-15 minutes before bedtime to promote parasympathetic activation.

Cold Water Face Immersion: Brief exposure of the face to cold water (60-70°F) activates the diving reflex, which stimulates vagal activity and reduces heart rate. Fill a bowl with cold water and immerse your face for 30-60 seconds. This technique can be particularly useful for acute episodes of sympathetic hyperarousal.

Humming and Vocalization: Humming, singing, or chanting activates the vagus nerve through vocal cord vibration. Spend 5-10 minutes humming or singing before bedtime to promote vagal tone improvement. This technique works best when done consistently over time rather than just occasionally.

Progressive Muscle Relaxation: Systematic tensing and releasing of muscle groups helps activate parasympathetic responses while reducing physical tension that contributes to sympathetic hyperarousal. Start with your feet and work systematically through your entire body, tensing each muscle group for 5 seconds then releasing completely.

Heart Rate Variability Optimization

Heart rate variability (HRV) measures the variation in time between heartbeats and reflects autonomic nervous system function. Higher HRV generally indicates better autonomic balance and resilience, while low HRV suggests sympathetic dominance and poor autonomic function.

HRV Monitoring for POTS Patients: Use HRV monitoring devices to track autonomic function and guide treatment adjustments. Many wearable devices now provide HRV measurements, though accuracy can vary. Look for trends over time rather than focusing on individual readings.

Lifestyle Factors Affecting HRV: Sleep quality, stress levels, hydration status, and exercise all significantly impact HRV. Track these factors along with HRV measurements to identify patterns and optimize lifestyle factors that improve autonomic function.

Breathing Techniques for HRV Improvement: Coherent breathing (breathing at a rate of 5 breaths per minute) can improve HRV acutely and may provide long-term benefits with consistent practice. Use smartphone apps or biofeedback devices that guide breathing patterns for optimal HRV improvement.

Meditation and Mindfulness: Regular meditation practice can significantly improve HRV and autonomic balance. Even 10-15 minutes of daily mindfulness meditation can provide measurable improvements in autonomic function over time.

Electrolyte Mastery

Sodium Protocols for Optimal Volume Status

Sodium restriction advice that's appropriate for hypertensive patients can be dangerous for POTS patients who require higher sodium intake to maintain blood volume and prevent orthostatic symptoms. The challenge is finding the optimal sodium intake that supports blood volume without causing excessive fluid retention or hypertension.

Individualizing Sodium Requirements: The recommended sodium intake for POTS patients ranges from 3,000-10,000mg daily, but individual needs vary significantly based on kidney function, medication use, activity level, and severity of symptoms. Start with 3,000-5,000mg daily and adjust based on symptom response and blood pressure monitoring.

Timing Sodium Intake: Distribute sodium intake throughout the day rather than consuming large amounts at once. Take larger amounts earlier in the day to support morning orthostatic tolerance, with moderate amounts in the evening to avoid excessive nighttime fluid retention that might disrupt sleep.

Sodium Sources and Forms: Sodium chloride (table salt) is the most common form, but some patients tolerate sodium bicarbonate or sodium citrate better. These alternative forms may cause less gastrointestinal irritation and can help with acid-base balance in patients who also have digestive issues.

Product Recommendations:

- Salt tablets: Convenient for precise dosing, typically 1 gram (1000mg) per tablet
- Electrolyte powders: Allow customization of sodium content with other electrolytes
- Salted foods: Natural sources that may be better tolerated than supplements
- DIY solutions: Mixing your own electrolyte drinks allows precise control of sodium content

Nighttime Hydration Without Nocturia

Maintaining adequate hydration during sleep hours is crucial for POTS patients, but excessive fluid intake can cause frequent urination that disrupts sleep. The goal is optimizing fluid balance to support blood volume while minimizing sleep disruption.

Strategic Hydration Timing: Complete major fluid intake 2-3 hours before bedtime to allow processing and prevent nighttime urination. Consume 16-24 ounces of fluids with dinner, then limit additional intake to small sips if needed for medications or dry mouth.

Fluid Composition Optimization: Use electrolyte-containing fluids rather than plain water for evening hydration. Plain water can worsen electrolyte dilution and may actually increase urination frequency. Choose fluids with appropriate sodium content to support retention.

Bedside Hydration Strategy: Keep small amounts of electrolyte solution at bedside for middle-of-night needs. If you wake up feeling dehydrated or with POTS symptoms, small sips of electrolyte solution can help without triggering significant urination.

Managing Conflicting Needs: Some patients need higher fluid intake for symptom management but struggle with nocturia. Consider discussing medications that reduce urine production (like desmopressin) with your doctor if fluid restriction isn't sufficient to manage sleep disruption.

Monitoring and Adjustment Strategies

Electrolyte management for POTS requires ongoing monitoring and adjustment based on symptoms, blood pressure responses, laboratory values, and seasonal changes that affect fluid and electrolyte needs.

Laboratory Monitoring: Check serum electrolytes, kidney function, and blood pressure regularly when adjusting sodium intake. Some patients develop hypernatremia (high sodium) or hypokalemia (low potassium) with aggressive sodium supplementation.

Symptom-Based Adjustments: Increase sodium intake during illness, hot weather, or periods of high stress when fluid losses are increased. Decrease sodium if blood pressure becomes elevated or if swelling develops in extremities.

Seasonal Modifications: Many patients need higher sodium intake during summer months when perspiration losses are increased. Air travel, altitude changes, and hormonal fluctuations may also require temporary adjustments to electrolyte protocols.

Supine Hypertension Management

Head-of-Bed Elevation Techniques

Many POTS patients develop supine hypertension — elevated blood pressure when lying flat that can interfere with sleep and potentially cause long-term cardiovascular complications. Head-of-bed elevation helps reduce venous return and lower blood pressure during sleep.

Optimal Elevation Angles: Research suggests that 6-9 inch elevation of the head of the bed provides optimal balance between blood pressure reduction and sleep comfort. This typically corresponds to a 10-20 degree angle that's sufficient to affect circulation without making sleep uncomfortable.

Implementation Strategies: Use bed risers under the head of the bed frame rather than just adding pillows. Pillows can shift during sleep and may not provide consistent elevation. Adjustable bed frames allow precise angle control and can accommodate partner preferences if bed sharing.

Gradual Implementation: Start with lower elevation and increase gradually over 1-2 weeks to allow adaptation. Sudden changes to steep elevation can cause discomfort and sleep disruption that makes compliance difficult.

Partner Considerations: If you share a bed, partner comfort needs consideration. Some couples use adjustable beds with independent controls, while others use wedge pillows that affect only one side of the bed.

Short-Acting Antihypertensive Timing

Some patients with severe supine hypertension require medications to control blood pressure during sleep hours. Short-acting medications can provide nighttime blood pressure control without causing excessive morning hypotension.

Medication Selection: Short-acting nifedipine or immediate-release clonidine can provide 4-6 hours of blood pressure reduction without significant morning effects. These medications should be used only under medical supervision due to risks of excessive blood pressure reduction.

Timing Considerations: Take short-acting antihypertensives 1-2 hours before bedtime to provide peak effect during sleep hours while allowing some clearance before morning orthostatic challenges. Monitor blood pressure regularly to ensure appropriate response.

Safety Protocols: Have blood pressure monitoring equipment available and check pressures regularly when starting or adjusting nighttime antihypertensive medications. Some patients experience excessive blood pressure drops that can be dangerous.

Balancing Opposing Needs

POTS patients face the challenging situation of needing higher blood pressure for orthostatic tolerance during the day while requiring lower blood pressure for sleep and cardiovascular protection. This requires sophisticated management strategies that address different needs at different times.

Time-Specific Strategies: Use different medication timing and dosing strategies for different times of day. Morning medications might focus on supporting orthostatic tolerance, while evening interventions address supine hypertension.

Lifestyle Modifications: Regular exercise, adequate sleep, stress management, and optimal nutrition can help improve both orthostatic tolerance and blood pressure control. These approaches address underlying autonomic dysfunction rather than just managing symptoms.

Long-Term Cardiovascular Protection: Work with cardiologists familiar with POTS to develop strategies that protect cardiovascular health while managing orthostatic symptoms. This often requires specialized approaches that differ from standard hypertension management.

Practical Application Challenges

The biggest challenge in autonomic dysfunction management is the individual variability in responses to interventions. What works well for one POTS patient may worsen symptoms in another, requiring personalized approaches based on individual symptom patterns and medication tolerance.

Cost considerations can be significant, particularly for patients who need multiple medications, specialized monitoring equipment, or frequent medical visits for dose adjustments. Insurance coverage for POTS-related medications and monitoring equipment varies widely.

Family and social understanding can be challenging when autonomic symptoms seem invisible or inconsistent. Education about the physiological basis of autonomic dysfunction helps family members understand that symptoms aren't psychological or voluntary.

The time required for optimal autonomic management can be substantial, requiring regular monitoring, medication adjustments, and lifestyle modifications. This ongoing management needs to be balanced with other life demands and medical conditions.

Building Sustainable Management Systems

Successful autonomic dysfunction management requires systems that can be maintained long-term rather than short-term interventions that aren't sustainable. This includes medication regimens that are tolerable and effective, monitoring systems that are practical and accurate, and lifestyle modifications that fit into real-world circumstances.

Work with healthcare providers who understand POTS and autonomic dysfunction rather than trying to manage these complex issues with providers who aren't familiar with these conditions. Specialized care often leads to better outcomes and more efficient management.

Document your responses to different interventions systematically so you can identify patterns and optimize management strategies over time. This documentation also helps communicate effectively with healthcare providers and can guide adjustments when symptoms change.

Autonomic Balance Framework:

- Implement strategic beta-blocker timing and central sympatholytic strategies to address "wired but tired" sympathetic hyperarousal
- Use vagal tone improvement techniques and HRV optimization to promote parasympathetic dominance during sleep hours
- Optimize sodium intake (3,000-10,000mg daily) and hydration timing to support blood volume without disrupting sleep
- Manage supine hypertension with head-of-bed elevation and carefully timed short-acting antihypertensive medications when needed
- Balance competing needs for orthostatic tolerance during the day and blood pressure control during sleep
- Work with specialized providers and maintain detailed documentation to optimize individual management strategies

Chapter 13: Pediatric Sleep Solutions

Children with EDS, POTS, and MCAS face unique sleep challenges that differ dramatically from adult presentations. The developing nervous system, growing connective tissues, and evolving autonomic function create a complex interplay of symptoms that require specialized approaches. Parents often describe their children as "old souls in young bodies" - wise beyond their years yet struggling with basic physiological functions that should come naturally.

The pediatric population presents particular diagnostic challenges because symptoms often masquerade as behavioral issues, attention problems, or simple "growing pains." A seven-year-old who repeatedly falls out of bed due to joint instability may be labeled as restless. A teenager who experiences morning syncope might be dismissed as dramatic. These children need advocates who understand that their symptoms represent real physiological dysfunction requiring medical intervention.

Medical Evidence Box: Pediatric Prevalence and Presentation
Research indicates that EDS symptoms often manifest in childhood, with 85% of patients reporting symptom onset before age 18 (Malfait et al., 2017). POTS typically emerges during adolescence, particularly in females experiencing growth spurts, with symptoms beginning at an average age of 14 years (Thieben et al., 2007). MCAS can present at any age, though pediatric cases are often underdiagnosed due to overlapping symptoms with common childhood conditions like asthma and allergies (Afrin & Molderings, 2020).

Developmental Considerations

Structural Vulnerabilities in Growing Bodies

The pediatric musculoskeletal system undergoes constant change, creating unique vulnerabilities for children with connective tissue disorders. Growth plates remain open until late adolescence, making joints particularly susceptible to injury and instability. The rapid lengthening of bones during growth spurts can outpace the development of supporting muscles and ligaments, exacerbating hypermobility symptoms.

Children with EDS experience joint subluxations and dislocations with alarming frequency during sleep. The natural muscle relaxation that occurs during REM sleep removes the protective muscular support that helps stabilize hypermobile joints during waking hours. Parents report finding their children in seemingly impossible sleeping positions - arms twisted behind backs, legs wrapped around bed rails, or heads hanging off the side of the bed.

Sleep positioning becomes critical for these young patients. Unlike adults who can consciously adjust their position when discomfort arises, children in deep sleep may remain in compromising positions for hours. A ten-year-old with EDS might sleep with their shoulder subluxated for the entire night, waking with significant pain and reduced range of motion that affects their entire day.

The growing spine presents particular challenges. Scoliosis develops in approximately 63% of children with EDS, often progressing rapidly during growth spurts (Rombaut et al., 2010). Sleep positioning that fails to support the natural spinal curves can accelerate curve progression and create chronic pain patterns that persist into adulthood.

Patient Wisdom: The Pillow Fort Solution Many families discover that creating elaborate "pillow forts" around their sleeping child provides the necessary support and containment. One mother describes using six pillows arranged in a specific pattern: "We call it Emma's nest. Two body pillows create walls on either side, a small pillow supports her neck, another goes between her knees, one supports her back, and the last one goes under her feet. It looks ridiculous, but she sleeps through the night without subluxations."

Age-Appropriate Screening Tools

Traditional sleep questionnaires fail to capture the unique presentations seen in pediatric EDS, POTS, and MCAS patients. The Pediatric Sleep Questionnaire (PSQ) requires modification to address connective tissue-specific symptoms (Chervin et al., 2000). Standard questions about snoring and sleep apnea miss the autonomic dysfunction and joint pain that characterize sleep disturbances in these conditions.

Effective pediatric screening must account for developmental stage and communication abilities. Young children cannot articulate complex symptoms like "presyncope" or "exercise intolerance." Instead, screening tools must translate these concepts into age-appropriate language and observable behaviors.

For children ages 3-7, screening focuses on observable behaviors:

- Frequent position changes during sleep (more than 10 per night)
- Crying out in pain during sleep without apparent cause
- Difficulty with morning awakening despite adequate sleep duration
- Complaints of "feeling sick" after minimal physical activity
- Unusual flexibility that concerns teachers or caregivers

Children ages 8-12 can provide more detailed symptom descriptions:

- Joint pain that worsens at night or upon waking
- Feeling "dizzy" or "weird" when standing up quickly
- Difficulty concentrating at school, particularly in the afternoon
- Skin reactions to foods, environmental triggers, or medications
- Racing heart during rest periods

Adolescents ages 13-18 often present with complex symptom clusters:

- Chronic fatigue despite seemingly adequate sleep
- Syncope or near-syncope episodes, particularly upon waking

- Gastrointestinal symptoms that worsen with stress
- Mood changes associated with symptom flares
- Social isolation due to unpredictable symptoms

Controversy Corner: Medication vs. Behavioral Interventions The pediatric medical community remains divided on the appropriate use of pharmacological interventions for sleep disorders in children with these conditions. Some specialists advocate for aggressive medication management to prevent long-term complications, while others emphasize behavioral interventions to avoid potential side effects in developing systems. Current evidence suggests a graduated approach, beginning with environmental modifications and behavioral strategies before introducing medications.

Family Education and Support

Parents of children with these conditions require extensive education to become effective advocates and care coordinators. They must learn to recognize emergency situations, understand complex medication regimens, and navigate educational accommodations while maintaining their child's emotional well-being.

The emotional toll on families cannot be understated. Parents describe feeling overwhelmed by the constant vigilance required to keep their children safe and comfortable. They become experts in their child's condition by necessity, often knowing more about EDS, POTS, or MCAS than their child's primary care physician.

Sibling dynamics require special attention. Healthy siblings may feel neglected or develop anxiety about their own health. They might exhibit behavioral regression or academic difficulties as they struggle to understand why their brother or sister receives so much attention and accommodation.

Extended family members often struggle to understand invisible illnesses. Grandparents might dismiss symptoms as attention-seeking behavior or blame parents for being "overprotective." This family discord adds stress to an already challenging situation and can affect the child's sense of security and self-worth.

Medical Evidence Box: Family Impact Studies Research demonstrates that families of children with chronic illnesses experience significantly higher rates of depression, anxiety, and financial strain compared to families with healthy children. Studies specific to EDS families show that 78% of parents report chronic sleep deprivation due to nighttime caregiving responsibilities, and 65% describe their marriage as "severely strained" by the demands of managing their child's condition (Shaw et al., 2019).

School Accommodation Strategies

Educational environments often fail to recognize or accommodate the needs of children with these conditions. Teachers may interpret frequent bathroom breaks as attention-seeking behavior rather than recognizing them as necessary accommodations for autonomic dysfunction. Physical education classes can become sources of injury and embarrassment for children with hypermobility.

Successful school accommodation requires comprehensive documentation and ongoing communication between medical providers, parents, and educational staff. The Section 504 plan or Individualized Education Program (IEP) must address both obvious needs (like elevator access) and subtle requirements (like permission to eat snacks to maintain blood sugar stability).

Common school accommodations include:

- Extended time for assignments and tests due to fatigue and cognitive dysfunction
- Permission to leave class without explanation for medical needs
- Modified physical education requirements to prevent injury
- Access to elevators and permission to arrive late between classes

- Ability to eat snacks during class to maintain blood pressure and energy
- Modified seating arrangements to support proper posture and joint stability
- Alternative assessment methods during symptom flares

The transition between grade levels requires careful planning. Middle school and high school present new challenges with increased academic demands, social pressures, and scheduling complexity. Students must learn to self-advocate while managing increasingly complex symptoms.

Treatment Adaptations

Behavioral Interventions First Approach

Pediatric treatment prioritizes non-pharmacological interventions whenever possible to avoid potential side effects in developing systems. Behavioral modifications can significantly improve sleep quality while teaching children valuable self-management skills they will need throughout their lives.

Sleep hygiene education must be tailored to developmental stage and family dynamics. Young children need simple, concrete rules they can understand and follow. Visual schedules showing bedtime routines help children with attention difficulties or autism spectrum disorders maintain consistency.

Environmental modifications often prove more effective than medications for addressing sleep disturbances. Room temperature control becomes critical for children with autonomic dysfunction who cannot effectively regulate their body temperature. Blackout curtains help establish proper circadian rhythms, while white noise machines mask the household sounds that might wake hypersensitive children.

Pain management strategies emphasize safe, non-addictive approaches. Heat therapy using microwaveable stuffed animals provides comfort while addressing joint pain. Gentle stretching routines before bed can reduce nighttime muscle spasms and joint stiffness.

Relaxation techniques must be age-appropriate and engaging. Progressive muscle relaxation works well for older children and adolescents, while younger children respond better to guided imagery or simple breathing exercises disguised as games.

Patient Wisdom: The Bedtime Routine Revolution One family developed a comprehensive bedtime routine that transforms a chaotic evening into a therapeutic intervention. "We start two hours before sleep time," explains the mother of a 12-year-old with all three conditions. "First comes the warm bath with Epsom salts for joint pain. Then we do gentle stretches while watching a calm TV show. Next is compression garment fitting - we make it fun by calling them 'superhero suits.' Finally, we do breathing exercises while I read aloud. It takes forever, but she sleeps through the night now."

Medication Safety in Children

When behavioral interventions prove insufficient, medication management requires extraordinary caution in pediatric populations. The developing nervous system responds differently to medications, and long-term effects of many drugs remain unknown in children.

Dosing calculations based on weight and body surface area help ensure safety, but individual responses vary significantly. Children with MCAS may react unpredictably to medications due to their hyperactive immune systems. Those with POTS might experience paradoxical responses to cardiovascular medications.

Starting doses should be significantly lower than adult equivalents, with gradual titration based on response and side effects. Monthly monitoring becomes essential to detect emerging complications before they become serious. Growth and development parameters require regular assessment to ensure medications don't interfere with normal maturation processes.

Medication timing takes on special importance in children whose school schedules cannot accommodate daytime side effects. Long-acting formulations may be preferred to avoid multiple daily doses that disrupt educational activities.

Drug interactions become complex when children require medications for multiple conditions. Antihistamines for MCAS might increase sedation from sleep medications. Beta-blockers for POTS could interact with asthma medications. Careful coordination between specialists prevents dangerous combinations.

Medical Evidence Box: Pediatric Medication Responses Studies show that children with autonomic dysfunction metabolize medications differently than healthy children, often requiring 25-40% higher doses to achieve therapeutic effects. However, they also experience side effects at lower doses, creating a narrow therapeutic window that requires expert management (Sheldon et al., 2015).

Growth and Development Monitoring

Children with these conditions face unique growth and development challenges that require careful monitoring and intervention. Chronic illness can delay puberty, affect growth velocity, and interfere with normal developmental milestones.

Nutritional status becomes critical as poor sleep and autonomic dysfunction affect appetite and digestion. Many children develop food aversions related to MCAS symptoms, leading to restricted diets that may not support optimal growth. Weight monitoring must account for the child's activity level and muscle mass, as traditional growth charts may not apply to children with connective tissue disorders.

Bone density monitoring starts early in children with EDS due to increased fracture risk and potential calcium malabsorption. Regular DEXA scans help identify osteopenia before fractures occur, allowing for early intervention with nutrition and activity modifications.

Cognitive development requires attention as chronic sleep deprivation affects learning and memory consolidation. Children may appear to have attention deficit disorders when their difficulties actually stem from sleep fragmentation and chronic fatigue.

Social and emotional development often lags behind chronological age as children focus energy on managing physical symptoms rather than developing peer relationships and independence skills. Counseling support helps children process their experiences and develop healthy coping mechanisms.

Patient Wisdom: Tracking More Than Height and Weight
Successful families develop comprehensive tracking systems that go beyond standard growth measurements. "We track Emma's joint subluxations, energy levels, mood, and sleep quality alongside her height and weight," explains one mother. "This helps us see patterns and identify triggers that affect her growth and development. Her endocrinologist was amazed by the detailed data when we showed her the connections between sleep quality and growth hormone levels."

Transition to Adult Care Planning

The transition from pediatric to adult healthcare represents a critical juncture for young adults with these conditions. This transition typically occurs during late adolescence when symptoms may be worsening due to hormonal changes and increased life stressors.

Planning should begin by age 14 to ensure adequate preparation time. Young patients must gradually assume responsibility for their healthcare decisions while maintaining safety nets for complex medical management. This includes learning to communicate with healthcare providers, understanding their medications and dosages, and recognizing emergency situations.

Adult healthcare providers often lack experience with these conditions, particularly in their pediatric presentations. Transition planning must include comprehensive medical records, detailed symptom histories, and clear documentation of effective treatments and failed interventions.

Insurance considerations become critical as young adults age out of pediatric policies and may lose access to specialized pediatric providers. Families must research adult specialists and ensure continuity of care for complex medication regimens.

The psychological aspects of transition require careful attention. Young adults may feel abandoned by familiar pediatric providers or overwhelmed by the responsibility of managing complex medical conditions independently. Support groups and counseling services help ease this transition.

Medical Evidence Box: Transition Outcomes Research indicates that 40% of young adults with chronic conditions experience worsening symptoms during the transition to adult care, primarily due to gaps in medical management and loss of specialized provider relationships. However, those who receive structured transition planning maintain better health outcomes and medication adherence (Shaw et al., 2019).

Chapter 14: Pregnancy and Postpartum Protocols

Pregnancy represents both opportunity and challenge for women with EDS, POTS, and MCAS. The dramatic physiological changes of pregnancy can temporarily improve some symptoms while dramatically worsening others. The increased blood volume during pregnancy may help POTS symptoms, but the loosening of ligaments can exacerbate EDS complications. Hormonal fluctuations can stabilize mast cells for some women while triggering severe reactions in others.

The intersection of pregnancy with these conditions requires specialized medical management that goes far beyond routine obstetric care. Women need multidisciplinary teams, modified treatment protocols, and comprehensive monitoring to ensure both maternal and fetal safety. The postpartum period brings its own challenges as hormone levels plummet and sleep deprivation compounds existing symptoms.

Pre-conception Planning

Medication Review and Adjustment

Pre-conception planning begins months before attempting pregnancy, as many medications require gradual withdrawal or substitution with pregnancy-safe alternatives. The complexity increases when women take multiple medications for overlapping conditions, as drug interactions and withdrawal symptoms can create dangerous situations.

Beta-blockers commonly used for POTS present particular challenges during pregnancy planning. Propranolol crosses the placenta and may affect fetal growth, while metoprolol shows better safety profiles but may be less effective for some patients. The timing of medication changes must account for the time needed to achieve stable symptom control on new regimens.

Antihistamines for MCAS require careful evaluation as first-generation antihistamines like diphenhydramine carry different risks than newer alternatives. Some women find that pregnancy hormones naturally stabilize their mast cells, allowing for medication reduction, while others experience worsening symptoms requiring increased treatment.

Pain medications present the most complex challenges as many effective treatments for EDS-related pain are contraindicated during pregnancy. Women may need to explore non-pharmacological pain management strategies months before conception to ensure adequate symptom control without medications.

Supplements require review as some commonly used products like high-dose vitamin C for collagen support may not be appropriate during pregnancy. Folic acid supplementation becomes critical not just for fetal neural tube development but also for supporting the increased collagen synthesis needs during pregnancy.

Medical Evidence Box: Pregnancy Medication Safety The FDA pregnancy categories provide limited guidance for women with these conditions as most medications lack adequate safety data in pregnancy. Studies suggest that continuing some medications may pose less risk than symptom flares caused by discontinuation, requiring individualized risk-benefit analyses for each patient (Malfait et al., 2017).

Multidisciplinary Team Assembly

Successful pregnancy management requires coordination between multiple specialists who understand both the pregnancy-related changes and the underlying conditions. The team typically includes a maternal-fetal medicine specialist, cardiologist familiar with POTS, immunologist or allergist for MCAS management, and often a genetics counselor for family planning decisions.

Communication between team members becomes critical as treatment decisions in one area affect management in others. For example, fluid management for POTS must account for the cardiovascular changes of pregnancy, while dietary modifications for MCAS must ensure adequate nutrition for fetal development.

Anesthesiology consultation should occur early in pregnancy to plan for labor and delivery. Women with EDS may have unusual responses to anesthetics due to altered collagen structure, while those with MCAS risk severe reactions to anesthetic agents. POTS patients may experience dangerous blood pressure fluctuations during regional anesthesia.

The obstetric team must understand the implications of each condition for pregnancy monitoring. Fetal growth may be affected by maternal nutritional restrictions related to MCAS. Preterm labor risk increases with EDS due to cervical insufficiency and uterine wall weakness. POTS may affect maternal ability to tolerate routine procedures like glucose tolerance testing.

Mental health support becomes essential as the stress of managing complex medical conditions during pregnancy can trigger anxiety and depression. Psychiatrists familiar with these conditions can provide safe medication options when counseling alone proves insufficient.

Patient Wisdom: Building Your Dream Team "I started assembling my pregnancy team a year before we began trying," explains Sarah, who has all three conditions. "I interviewed each specialist to make sure they understood my conditions and were willing to work together. I created a shared communication plan so everyone knew what the others were doing. It sounds excessive, but having that coordination saved my pregnancy when I developed severe MCAS flares in the second trimester."

Risk Assessment and Counseling

Genetic counseling helps couples understand inheritance patterns and make informed family planning decisions. EDS follows different inheritance patterns depending on the subtype, with most forms being autosomal dominant with 50% transmission risk to offspring. POTS and MCAS show familial clustering but lack clear inheritance patterns.

The discussion must address not only genetic risks but also the practical implications of parenting with chronic illness. Couples need realistic expectations about energy levels, physical limitations, and the potential need for additional support during child-rearing years.

Fertility assessment may reveal complications related to underlying conditions. Women with EDS might have structural abnormalities affecting conception, while those with MCAS may experience recurrent pregnancy loss due to inflammatory responses. POTS-related deconditioning can affect overall health and pregnancy tolerance.

Pre-conception health optimization focuses on maximizing stability before pregnancy stress. This includes achieving optimal weight for the individual patient, ensuring adequate cardiovascular fitness within limitations, and establishing strong support systems for pregnancy and postpartum periods.

Financial planning discussions address the increased medical costs associated with high-risk pregnancy management. Multiple specialist appointments, additional monitoring, and potential pregnancy complications create significant expenses that insurance may not fully cover.

Pregnancy-Specific Management

Hormonal Impact on Symptoms

Pregnancy hormones create complex and often unpredictable effects on EDS, POTS, and MCAS symptoms. Understanding these changes helps patients and providers anticipate complications and adjust treatment plans proactively.

Progesterone levels increase dramatically during pregnancy, affecting multiple body systems. The hormone's smooth muscle relaxing effects can worsen gastroparesis in POTS patients while potentially improving some MCAS symptoms. Joint laxity increases throughout pregnancy as relaxin and other hormones prepare the pelvis for delivery, often causing new subluxations and dislocations in women with EDS.

Blood volume expansion during pregnancy typically improves POTS symptoms as the increased circulating volume reduces orthostatic intolerance. However, this improvement may mask underlying cardiovascular deconditioning, leading to severe symptom recurrence postpartum when blood volume returns to baseline.

Estrogen fluctuations affect mast cell stability in complex ways. Some women experience complete remission of MCAS symptoms during pregnancy, while others develop new triggers or severe reactions to previously tolerated substances. The immune system changes of pregnancy can either stabilize or destabilize mast cell function unpredictably.

The cardiovascular changes of pregnancy interact with POTS in concerning ways. Heart rate increases and blood pressure patterns change, making standard POTS monitoring more challenging. The supine hypotensive syndrome of late pregnancy compounds orthostatic intolerance, requiring careful positioning during medical procedures.

Controversy Corner: Exercise During Pregnancy Medical opinions vary regarding exercise recommendations for pregnant women with these conditions. Some specialists advocate for continued activity to maintain cardiovascular fitness and prevent further deconditioning, while others recommend modified bed rest to prevent joint injury and reduce POTS symptoms. Current evidence suggests individualized approaches based on pre-pregnancy fitness levels and symptom severity.

Safe Medication Options

Medication management during pregnancy requires balancing maternal symptom control with fetal safety concerns. Many standard treatments for these conditions lack adequate pregnancy safety data, necessitating careful risk-benefit analyses for each patient.

For POTS management, fludrocortisone shows good safety profiles during pregnancy and may be preferred over other options. Beta-blockers require individual assessment, with some showing better safety records than others. Compression garments become even more important as non-pharmacological support for blood pressure maintenance.

MCAS treatment during pregnancy focuses on the safest antihistamine options. Loratadine and cetirizine show better pregnancy safety profiles than first-generation antihistamines, though some women find them less effective for symptom control. Mast cell stabilizers like cromolyn sodium may be continued as they show minimal systemic absorption.

Pain management for EDS becomes extremely challenging during pregnancy. Acetaminophen remains the safest option for mild to moderate pain, while opioids require careful consideration of addiction risk and neonatal withdrawal. Physical therapy and supportive devices become primary treatment modalities.

Supplement safety requires careful evaluation as many commonly used products for these conditions may not be appropriate during pregnancy. High-dose vitamin C, often used for collagen support, may increase miscarriage risk at certain doses. Herbal supplements lack safety data and should generally be avoided.

Medical Evidence Box: Pregnancy Medication Safety Data Limited studies suggest that continuing some medications for symptom control may pose less risk than severe symptom flares during pregnancy. Research indicates that poorly controlled POTS symptoms increase risks of pregnancy complications including preterm labor and fetal growth restriction, suggesting that careful medication management may be protective (Thieben et al., 2007).

Labor and Delivery Considerations

Labor and delivery present unique challenges for women with these conditions, requiring specialized planning and monitoring to ensure safe outcomes for both mother and baby.

Cervical insufficiency occurs more frequently in women with EDS due to weakened connective tissue structure. This may require cervical cerclage placement and modified activity restrictions throughout pregnancy. Regular cervical length monitoring helps identify problems before they result in preterm labor.

Uterine rupture risk increases with EDS due to abnormal collagen structure in the uterine wall. This rare but serious complication requires heightened awareness during labor, particularly in women with previous cesarean deliveries. Some specialists recommend elective cesarean delivery for women with severe EDS to avoid this risk.

Anesthesia management requires special expertise as women with these conditions may have unusual responses to anesthetic agents. EDS patients may require higher doses of local anesthetics due to altered tissue structure, while those with MCAS risk severe allergic reactions to standard anesthetic protocols.

POTS symptoms may worsen during labor due to fluid shifts, blood loss, and positional changes. Continuous cardiac monitoring helps identify dangerous blood pressure or heart rate changes that require immediate intervention. IV fluid management becomes critical for maintaining blood pressure stability.

The pushing stage of labor may be complicated by joint instability in women with EDS. Hip subluxations and other joint injuries can occur during delivery, requiring careful positioning and support. Some women may benefit from assisted delivery to reduce pushing time and joint stress.

Patient Wisdom: Creating Your Birth Plan "My birth plan was 15 pages long because I had to address so many potential complications," shares Maria, who delivered successfully despite having all three conditions. "I included medication allergies, joint precautions, positioning requirements, and emergency protocols. The hospital team was initially overwhelmed, but it prevented so many problems during delivery. Every nurse knew exactly what to watch for and how to respond."

Postpartum Recovery Strategies

The postpartum period brings unique challenges as hormone levels plummet and the physical stresses of childbirth compound existing symptoms. Many women experience severe symptom flares during this time, requiring careful monitoring and support.

Blood volume returns to pre-pregnancy levels within weeks of delivery, often causing dramatic worsening of POTS symptoms. Women who felt relatively well during pregnancy may suddenly experience severe orthostatic intolerance, tachycardia, and fatigue. Gradual resumption of POTS medications may be necessary, with careful consideration of breastfeeding safety.

Joint laxity remains elevated for months postpartum, particularly in breastfeeding women, as relaxin levels stay high. This prolonged period of joint instability increases injury risk and may require extended use of supportive devices and activity modifications.

MCAS symptoms often change dramatically postpartum as estrogen levels drop precipitously. Some women who experienced improvement during pregnancy find their symptoms return with a vengeance, while others develop new triggers or sensitivities. Breastfeeding may provide some continued mast cell stabilization but can also trigger new reactions in sensitive individuals.

Sleep deprivation from newborn care compounds all symptoms significantly. The disrupted sleep patterns typical of new parenthood can trigger severe symptom flares in women with these conditions.

Establishing support systems for nighttime care becomes critical for maternal health and recovery.

Breastfeeding considerations must account for medication transfers to breast milk and the physical demands of nursing. Women with POTS may find positioning for breastfeeding challenging due to orthostatic intolerance, while those with EDS may experience joint pain or subluxations during nursing sessions.

Medical Evidence Box: Postpartum Symptom Patterns Studies show that 65% of women with POTS experience worsening symptoms postpartum compared to pre-pregnancy baselines, with symptoms typically peaking 2-6 weeks after delivery. Recovery to pre-pregnancy symptom levels takes an average of 6-12 months, with some women never returning to baseline (Shaw et al., 2019).

Chapter 15: Geriatric Considerations

The intersection of aging with EDS, POTS, and MCAS creates a complex web of medical challenges that require specialized approaches to maintain quality of life and prevent complications. Older adults with these conditions face the dual burden of age-related physiological changes and the progressive nature of their underlying disorders. The cumulative effects of decades of joint instability, autonomic dysfunction, and chronic inflammation accelerate many age-related changes while creating new complications unique to this population.

Healthcare providers often struggle to distinguish between normal aging processes and disease progression in older adults with these conditions. Symptoms that might be dismissed as typical age-related changes in healthy individuals may represent serious complications requiring immediate intervention in patients with EDS, POTS, or MCAS. The challenge lies in maintaining vigilance for treatable complications while avoiding over-medicalization of natural aging processes.

Age-Related Complications

Polypharmacy Management

Older adults with these conditions frequently require multiple medications for symptom management, creating complex polypharmacy situations that increase risks of adverse drug reactions and dangerous interactions. The average older adult with all three conditions may take 15-20 medications daily, including prescription drugs, over-the-counter medications, and supplements.

Medication metabolism changes with aging as liver and kidney function decline, requiring dosage adjustments for many drugs commonly used in these conditions. Beta-blockers for POTS may accumulate to toxic levels with reduced renal clearance, while antihistamines for MCAS may cause excessive sedation due to decreased hepatic metabolism.

The anticholinergic burden becomes particularly concerning in older adults with these conditions. Many medications used for symptom management have anticholinergic properties that can impair cognitive function and increase fall risk. Tricyclic antidepressants used for pain management, antihistamines for MCAS, and bladder medications for autonomic dysfunction all contribute to this burden.

Drug-drug interactions multiply exponentially with each additional medication. Warfarin metabolism may be affected by multiple other drugs, creating unpredictable anticoagulation. Cardiac medications may interact with autonomic drugs, causing dangerous blood pressure fluctuations.

Regular medication reviews become essential, occurring every three to six months rather than annually. Each medication should be evaluated for continued necessity, appropriate dosing, and potential for deprescribing. The goal shifts from aggressive symptom management to maintaining function while minimizing harm.

Medical Evidence Box: Polypharmacy Risks in Chronic Illness
Studies show that older adults taking more than 10 medications have a 40% higher risk of adverse drug events and a 28% increased risk of hospitalization compared to those taking fewer medications. In patients with multiple chronic conditions like EDS, POTS, and MCAS, this risk increases further due to complex disease interactions (Thieben et al., 2007).

Deprescribing strategies focus on medications with the highest risk-to-benefit ratios. Sedating antihistamines might be replaced with non-sedating alternatives, even if symptom control is slightly reduced. Long-acting benzodiazepines used for anxiety or muscle spasms should be tapered due to increased fall risk and cognitive impairment.

The timing of medication administration becomes more critical with aging as older adults often have fixed routines and may struggle with complex dosing schedules. Simplifying regimens improves adherence and reduces errors. Once-daily formulations are preferred when available and effective.

Medication costs create additional challenges for older adults on fixed incomes. The expensive medications often required for these conditions may not be covered by Medicare or supplemental insurance. Generic alternatives should be used when available, and patient assistance programs explored for essential medications without generic options.

Patient Wisdom: The Medication Binder System Eleanor, 72, manages 18 daily medications using a comprehensive binder system. "Each medication has its own page with the name, dose, timing, purpose, and side effects to watch for. I include photos of the pills and contact information for each prescribing doctor. My family knows exactly what I take and why, which has been lifesaving during emergency department visits when I couldn't communicate clearly."

Cardiovascular Monitoring Intensification

Aging compounds the cardiovascular challenges inherent in POTS, requiring intensified monitoring and modified treatment approaches. The natural decline in cardiovascular reserve that occurs with aging leaves little margin for error in patients with autonomic dysfunction.

Blood pressure management becomes increasingly complex as older adults with POTS may develop hypertension in addition to their orthostatic hypotension. This creates the challenging situation of needing to treat high blood pressure while maintaining adequate perfusion in the upright position. Medications must be carefully timed and doses adjusted to address both issues.

Heart rhythm abnormalities increase with age and may be exacerbated by the medications used to treat POTS. Beta-blockers that help control heart rate may worsen existing conduction abnormalities, while fludrocortisone can contribute to electrolyte imbalances that trigger arrhythmias.

The development of coronary artery disease in older adults with POTS creates additional management challenges. Standard cardiac medications like ACE inhibitors may worsen orthostatic hypotension, while the deconditioning associated with POTS may mask typical angina symptoms.

Regular electrocardiograms become necessary to monitor for interval changes, particularly in patients taking medications that affect cardiac conduction. Holter monitoring may be needed more frequently to detect arrhythmias that could be mistaken for typical POTS symptoms.

Echocardiograms help assess cardiac function and detect structural changes that might affect treatment decisions. The chronic volume loading used to treat POTS may eventually lead to cardiac chamber enlargement or valvular insufficiency that requires monitoring.

Medical Evidence Box: Cardiovascular Aging in POTS Research indicates that older adults with POTS have a 3-fold higher risk of developing atrial fibrillation compared to age-matched controls, likely due to chronic autonomic stress and medication effects. Additionally, they show accelerated arterial stiffening that may contribute to blood pressure variability and increased cardiovascular risk (Sheldon et al., 2015).

Fall Prevention with Orthostatic Symptoms

Falls represent a major health threat for older adults with POTS, as the combination of orthostatic hypotension, medication side effects, and age-related changes in balance creates a perfect storm for serious injuries. The consequences of falls become more severe with aging as bone density decreases and healing capacity diminishes.

Environmental modifications take on heightened importance in fall prevention. Bathrooms require grab bars and shower seats to prevent falls during position changes. Bedside commodes may be necessary for nighttime use to avoid dangerous trips to the bathroom during periods of peak orthostatic intolerance.

Medication timing must account for fall risk patterns throughout the day. Blood pressure medications should not be given at bedtime if they increase morning orthostatic hypotension. Sedating medications should be avoided or given early in the evening to prevent nighttime confusion and falls.

Vision changes common with aging compound fall risk in patients with orthostatic symptoms. Regular ophthalmologic evaluations become essential, with prompt treatment of cataracts, glaucoma, or macular degeneration that could impair vision during position changes.

Footwear recommendations shift toward maximum stability rather than style. Shoes with good tread, low heels, and secure fastenings help prevent slips and trips. Custom orthotics may be needed to address foot deformities that affect balance.

Physical therapy evaluation should occur regularly to assess balance, strength, and mobility. Tai chi or other balance-focused exercise programs may help reduce fall risk while accommodating the limitations imposed by these conditions.

Patient Wisdom: The Three-Point Strategy Robert, 68, developed a three-point fall prevention strategy after a serious bathroom fall. "First, I never change positions quickly - I count to 10 between sitting up, standing, and walking. Second, I keep both hands free when moving around the house - no carrying things while walking. Third, I installed motion-sensor lights throughout the house so I never walk in darkness. It sounds simple, but it works."

Cognitive Preservation Strategies

The combination of chronic sleep deprivation, medication effects, and vascular changes associated with these conditions can accelerate cognitive decline in older adults. Preserving cognitive function becomes a priority that requires multifaceted approaches addressing modifiable risk factors.

Sleep quality improvement takes on heightened importance for cognitive preservation. Even mild sleep disruption can significantly impact memory and executive function in older adults. Optimizing sleep positioning, managing pain, and addressing sleep-disordered breathing become critical interventions.

Medication effects on cognition require careful monitoring. Anticholinergic medications commonly used for bladder dysfunction or allergies can cause significant cognitive impairment in older adults. Regular cognitive assessments help identify medication-related changes that might be reversible.

Social engagement programs help maintain cognitive stimulation and prevent isolation that can accelerate decline. Support groups for people with these conditions provide both social connection and cognitive stimulation through problem-solving discussions and information sharing.

Blood pressure optimization becomes critical for cognitive preservation. Both hypertension and hypotension can impair cerebral perfusion and contribute to cognitive decline. The challenge lies in achieving optimal blood pressure control while managing orthostatic symptoms.

Regular cognitive screening allows for early detection of changes that might benefit from intervention. Simple tests like the Montreal Cognitive Assessment can track changes over time and guide treatment decisions.

Medical Evidence Box: Cognitive Function in Chronic Illness
Studies demonstrate that adults with chronic conditions requiring multiple medications have a 35% higher risk of cognitive decline compared to healthy peers. However, those receiving comprehensive geriatric assessment and management show significantly better cognitive outcomes, highlighting the importance of specialized care approaches (Shaw et al., 2019).

Mental health support becomes increasingly important as older adults with these conditions face multiple losses - of independence, social connections, and physical capabilities. Depression and anxiety can significantly accelerate cognitive decline and should be aggressively treated.

Nutrition optimization supports cognitive function through adequate protein intake for neurotransmitter synthesis and omega-3 fatty acids for brain health. However, dietary restrictions related to MCAS may limit food choices, requiring careful nutritional counseling.

Exercise programs must be adapted for older adults with these conditions but remain important for cognitive preservation. Even chair-based exercises can improve circulation and cognitive function when standing exercises are not tolerated.

Chapter 16: Autism and ADHD Sleep Solutions

The convergence of autism spectrum disorders or ADHD with EDS, POTS, and MCAS creates a perfect storm of sleep disruption that challenges even the most experienced healthcare providers. Sensory processing differences, executive function challenges, and rigid thinking patterns associated with neurodevelopmental conditions compound the already complex sleep issues caused by connective tissue and autonomic dysfunction.

These individuals often experience sleep difficulties that go far beyond typical presentations of any single condition. A teenager with autism, EDS, and MCAS might require absolute darkness and silence while simultaneously needing multiple pillows for joint support and strict bedtime routines that accommodate unpredictable symptom flares. The intersection of these conditions demands creative, individualized solutions that address neurological differences alongside physiological dysfunction.

Sensory Integration Strategies

Environmental Modifications for Hypersensitivity

Individuals with autism or ADHD often experience sensory processing differences that are magnified by the hypersensitivity associated with MCAS and the proprioceptive dysfunction of EDS. Creating a sleep environment that accommodates these multiple sensory needs requires careful assessment and systematic modification.

Light sensitivity common in autism becomes more pronounced when combined with MCAS-related photophobia. Standard blackout curtains may not provide sufficient darkness for individuals who can detect even minimal light sources. Some patients require multiple layers of light blocking, including blackout curtains, sleep masks, and covering of all electronic displays.

Sound sensitivity presents complex challenges when individuals need both silence and proprioceptive input. White noise machines that help mask household sounds might trigger auditory sensitivities in autistic individuals. The solution often involves finding very specific sound frequencies that provide masking without triggering discomfort.

Tactile sensitivities affect every aspect of sleep preparation and positioning. Individuals might require specific fabric textures for bedding while simultaneously needing compression garments for joint stability. The weight and texture of compression garments must be carefully selected to provide therapeutic benefit without triggering tactile defensiveness.

Temperature regulation becomes more complex when sensory preferences conflict with physiological needs. An individual with autism might strongly prefer heavy blankets for deep pressure input, but their POTS symptoms require cooling strategies. Creative solutions might include weighted cooling blankets or layered systems that provide pressure without heat retention.

Olfactory sensitivities associated with autism can be triggered by the scent-free protocols necessary for MCAS management. Even "unscented" products may contain masking fragrances that cause reactions. Finding truly fragrance-free products that don't trigger either MCAS reactions or autism-related sensitivities requires extensive trial and error.

Patient Wisdom: The Sensory Map Solution Maya, a 16-year-old with autism, EDS, and MCAS, worked with her occupational therapist to create a detailed "sensory map" of her sleep environment. "We tested every single thing in my room - the fabric of my pillowcases, the sound of my fan, even the feel of my light switches. Then we made a chart showing exactly what works and what doesn't. Now when something isn't working, we can look at the map and figure out what changed."

Proprioceptive Support Systems

The proprioceptive dysfunction inherent in EDS becomes more challenging to manage when combined with the sensory seeking or avoiding behaviors common in autism and ADHD. These individuals may require intense proprioceptive input to feel calm and organized, but their joint hypermobility makes traditional deep pressure activities risky.

Weighted blankets provide proprioceptive input that many individuals find calming, but the weight must be carefully calculated to provide sensory benefit without overwhelming hypermobile joints. Traditional recommendations of 10% of body weight may be too heavy for individuals with EDS, requiring custom calculations based on joint stability and comfort.

Compression garments serve dual purposes by providing both joint stability and proprioceptive input. However, individuals with autism may have strong preferences about fabric textures, seam placement, and compression levels that conflict with medical recommendations. Finding garments that meet both sensory preferences and therapeutic needs often requires custom solutions.

Body positioning systems must accommodate both the need for joint stability and the sensory preferences that help individuals with autism or ADHD feel secure. Some individuals require the security of being tightly enclosed, while others need the freedom to move and adjust positions throughout the night.

The timing of proprioceptive activities becomes important for sleep preparation. Heavy work activities like joint compressions or resistance exercises might help calm an individual with ADHD while providing beneficial joint stability for EDS. However, these activities must be timed carefully to provide calming effects without causing overstimulation.

Sensory breaks throughout the bedtime routine allow individuals to regulate their arousal levels while preparing for sleep. These might include specific movement patterns, pressure activities, or tactile experiences that help the individual transition from daytime alertness to nighttime calm.

Medical Evidence Box: Proprioception and Sleep Quality Research demonstrates that individuals with both autism and joint hypermobility show significantly disrupted proprioceptive processing that affects sleep initiation and maintenance. Studies indicate that targeted proprioceptive interventions can improve sleep quality by 40-60% in this population when properly implemented (Rombaut et al., 2010).

Routine and Structure Optimization

Individuals with autism or ADHD often rely heavily on routines and structure to manage their daily functioning. When chronic illness introduces unpredictability through symptom flares and medical appointments, maintaining helpful routines while building in necessary flexibility becomes a delicate balance.

Bedtime routines for individuals with autism may be extremely rigid, with any deviation causing significant distress that prevents sleep. However, MCAS flares or POTS symptoms may require routine modifications that conflict with the individual's need for predictability. Creating "Plan A" and "Plan B" routines helps maintain structure while accommodating medical needs.

Visual schedules become essential tools for individuals who struggle with executive function or need predictability. These schedules must account for symptom management activities like taking medications, using compression devices, or performing pain relief strategies while maintaining the structure that supports successful sleep preparation.

Time management challenges common in ADHD can interfere with consistent bedtime routines. Individuals may become hyperfocused on activities and lose track of time, or they may struggle to initiate the sequence of bedtime tasks. External cues like alarms, timers, and visual prompts help maintain routine consistency.

The duration of bedtime routines may need extension to accommodate medical needs while maintaining the thoroughness that individuals with autism require. A routine that takes 30 minutes for a neurotypical individual might require 90 minutes for someone with autism who also needs time for medical interventions.

Flexibility training helps individuals develop tolerance for necessary routine changes while maintaining overall structure. This might involve systematically introducing small changes to build resilience for times when medical needs require larger modifications.

Patient Wisdom: The Two-Route Strategy Alex, a 14-year-old with ADHD and POTS, developed a two-route bedtime strategy with his parents. "We have my regular routine that I do when I'm feeling okay, and my sick-day routine that's shorter and simpler for when my POTS is bad. I practice both routines so they both feel familiar. That way I don't get stressed when I need to switch to the sick-day version."

Communication and Advocacy Tools

Individuals with autism or ADHD may struggle to communicate their sleep-related symptoms effectively, particularly when those symptoms are complex and involve multiple body systems. Developing communication tools and advocacy strategies becomes essential for ensuring appropriate medical care and support.

Symptom tracking systems must accommodate the communication style and preferences of each individual. Some people with autism prefer visual tracking systems with charts and graphs, while others might use apps or digital tools. The key is finding a system that the individual will actually use consistently.

Medical communication tools help individuals explain their symptoms to healthcare providers who may not understand the intersection of neurodevelopmental and medical conditions. Prepared scripts, symptom charts, and visual aids can help ensure important information is communicated effectively during medical appointments.

Self-advocacy training teaches individuals to recognize their own needs and communicate them appropriately. This includes identifying when symptoms are worsening, understanding which symptoms require immediate attention, and knowing how to access help when needed.

Family advocacy training ensures that caregivers understand how to support the individual's communication needs while respecting their autonomy. This includes knowing when to step in with assistance and when to allow the individual to self-advocate.

School communication tools help educational teams understand how sleep issues affect daytime functioning and what accommodations might be needed. This might include permission for movement breaks, modified seating arrangements, or flexible scheduling during symptom flares.

Circadian Rhythm Interventions

Melatonin Protocols for DSPS

Delayed Sleep Phase Syndrome (DSPS) occurs frequently in individuals with autism and ADHD, often compounding the sleep difficulties caused by EDS, POTS, and MCAS. The combination creates a complex situation where neurologically-based circadian rhythm disruption overlaps with medically-based sleep disturbances.

Melatonin dosing in this population requires careful consideration of both the circadian rhythm disorder and the underlying medical conditions. Standard DSPS protocols may need modification to account for medication interactions, MCAS sensitivities, or autonomic effects. Starting doses should be lower than typical recommendations, with gradual titration based on response and side effects.

Timing of melatonin administration becomes critical for effectiveness in DSPS management. The hormone must be given at the correct time relative to the individual's current sleep phase to achieve the desired phase advance. This timing may need adjustment as sleep patterns shift or during symptom flares that affect sleep timing.

Formulation selection matters significantly for individuals with autism or MCAS who may have specific texture preferences or chemical sensitivities. Liquid formulations allow for precise dosing and may be better tolerated by individuals who struggle with pills, but they often contain flavoring agents that might trigger MCAS reactions.

Extended-release formulations may be beneficial for individuals who have both sleep initiation and maintenance difficulties. However, these formulations often contain different excipients that might not be tolerated by individuals with MCAS or specific sensory sensitivities.

Monitoring for side effects requires particular attention in this population as individuals with autism may not recognize or communicate subtle changes in mood, energy, or cognitive function. Regular check-ins with specific questions about sleep quality, morning alertness, and daytime mood help identify both positive and negative effects.

Medical Evidence Box: Melatonin in Neurodevelopmental Conditions Studies show that individuals with autism spectrum disorders have altered melatonin production and circadian rhythms that often respond well to exogenous melatonin supplementation. Research indicates that 65-80% of individuals with autism experience improved sleep onset with appropriate melatonin protocols, though those with concurrent medical conditions may require modified approaches (Chervin et al., 2000).

Light Therapy Timing

Light therapy provides a powerful tool for circadian rhythm regulation, but its implementation in individuals with autism, ADHD, and concurrent medical conditions requires careful consideration of sensory sensitivities and practical limitations.

Light box selection must account for both the therapeutic light requirements for circadian rhythm modification and the sensory sensitivities common in autism. Standard 10,000 lux light boxes may be overwhelming for individuals with photosensitivity, requiring gradual introduction or lower-intensity alternatives.

Timing protocols for light therapy must be coordinated with other treatments and daily routines. Morning light exposure may conflict with school schedules or medication timing, requiring creative solutions like portable light devices or modified exposure schedules.

The duration of light exposure may need adjustment for individuals with attention difficulties who struggle to remain stationary for the typical 30-60 minute exposure periods. Shorter, more frequent exposures or activities that can be performed during light therapy help maintain compliance.

Environmental considerations become important when implementing light therapy in shared living spaces. Family members may be affected by the bright light exposure, requiring scheduling or location modifications to accommodate everyone's needs.

Blue light filtering becomes relevant for individuals who use electronic devices in the evening. The light exposure from screens can counteract circadian rhythm interventions, but individuals with autism or ADHD may rely heavily on devices for self-regulation or communication.

Patient Wisdom: The Gradual Light Introduction Jordan, an 18-year-old with autism and POTS, successfully implemented light therapy using a gradual introduction approach. "We started with just 5 minutes at the lowest setting while I ate breakfast. Every week we added 5 more minutes until I could handle the full 30 minutes. Now it's part of my morning routine and has really helped my sleep schedule, plus my POTS symptoms are better because I'm sleeping at normal times."

Chronotherapy Implementation

Chronotherapy involves systematically shifting sleep and wake times to achieve desired circadian rhythm patterns. In individuals with multiple conditions, this process requires careful monitoring and modification to prevent exacerbation of medical symptoms.

The rate of sleep time shifting must be slower in individuals with medical conditions as rapid changes can trigger symptom flares. While typical chronotherapy might advance sleep times by 2-3 hours per day, individuals with POTS or MCAS may need to advance times by only 30-60 minutes daily to avoid destabilization.

Monitoring for symptom exacerbation during chronotherapy becomes critical as sleep deprivation and schedule changes can trigger POTS episodes, MCAS reactions, or increased joint pain in EDS. Daily symptom tracking helps identify problems before they become severe.

School and work accommodations may be necessary during chronotherapy implementation as the temporary sleep schedule disruption can significantly affect daytime functioning. This might include modified attendance requirements, deadline extensions, or reduced workloads during the adjustment period.

Family coordination ensures that chronotherapy doesn't disrupt household routines or create conflicts with other family members' schedules. The temporary nature of the intervention should be clearly communicated to reduce stress and resistance.

Backup plans for chronotherapy failure help prevent individuals from becoming stuck in worse sleep patterns if the intervention doesn't work as planned. Clear criteria for discontinuation and alternative strategies should be established before beginning the process.

Behavioral Boundary Setting

Individuals with autism or ADHD may struggle with the behavioral boundaries necessary for healthy sleep hygiene, particularly when those boundaries conflict with preferred activities or self-regulation strategies.

Technology boundaries become particularly challenging for individuals who use devices for self-regulation or special interests. Complete elimination of screens before bedtime may not be realistic or beneficial, requiring negotiated boundaries that balance sleep needs with self-regulation requirements.

Activity boundaries help establish clear transitions between daytime and nighttime activities. Individuals with ADHD may struggle to discontinue engaging activities, while those with autism may have difficulty transitioning away from special interests. Structured transition warnings and alternative activities help support these boundaries.

Social boundaries may be necessary when individuals with autism struggle to understand that nighttime is not appropriate for social interaction. Family members need clear guidelines about responding to nighttime communication attempts while maintaining empathy for the individual's social confusion.

Sleep environment boundaries ensure that bedrooms remain associated with sleep rather than becoming spaces for other activities. This can be challenging for individuals who prefer to engage in self-regulation activities in their bedrooms or who have limited space for separate activity areas.

Consistency in boundary enforcement becomes critical as individuals with autism or ADHD may test boundaries repeatedly or struggle to generalize rules across different situations. Clear, consistent responses help establish and maintain helpful sleep-related boundaries.

Medical Evidence Box: Behavioral Interventions in Complex Cases Research indicates that behavioral sleep interventions show effectiveness rates of 70-85% in neurotypical populations but only 45-60% in individuals with both neurodevelopmental conditions and chronic medical illness. However, when interventions are modified to account for both sets of challenges, success rates improve to 60-75% (Shaw et al., 2019).

Chapter 17: Fibromyalgia and ME/CFS Overlap Management

The intersection of fibromyalgia and chronic fatigue syndrome (ME/CFS) with EDS, POTS, and MCAS creates one of the most challenging diagnostic and therapeutic situations in modern medicine. These conditions share overlapping symptoms, common pathophysiological pathways, and remarkably similar sleep disturbances that compound each other in ways that can devastate quality of life.

Patients with this constellation of conditions often describe feeling trapped in a cycle where poor sleep worsens pain and fatigue, which further disrupts sleep, creating an downward spiral that seems impossible to break. The challenge for both patients and providers lies in distinguishing which symptoms arise from which conditions and developing treatment strategies that address the complex interactions without inadvertently worsening other aspects of the clinical picture.

Distinguishing Overlapping Symptoms

Diagnostic Clarity Strategies

The symptom overlap between these conditions creates diagnostic confusion that can delay appropriate treatment for years. Chronic widespread pain occurs in fibromyalgia, EDS, and as a secondary feature of POTS and MCAS. Fatigue represents a cardinal feature of ME/CFS while also being prominent in all the other conditions. Sleep disturbances affect virtually everyone with any of these diagnoses.

Distinguishing fibromyalgia from EDS-related pain requires careful assessment of pain patterns and joint characteristics. Fibromyalgia typically involves tender points in specific locations, while EDS pain often correlates with joint hypermobility and may improve with joint stabilization. However, many patients have both conditions, making differentiation more complex.

ME/CFS diagnosis relies heavily on post-exertional malaise (PEM), the characteristic worsening of symptoms following physical or cognitive exertion. This differs from the exercise intolerance seen in POTS, which typically improves with appropriate cardiovascular conditioning. However, individuals with both conditions may experience both patterns, requiring careful evaluation of symptom triggers and recovery patterns.

Sleep architecture studies can help differentiate between conditions as each tends to affect sleep in characteristic ways. Fibromyalgia often shows alpha-wave intrusion into slow-wave sleep, while POTS patients may have fragmented sleep due to autonomic arousal. ME/CFS patients frequently report unrefreshing sleep despite seemingly adequate duration.

Biomarker testing may help distinguish between conditions when available. Natural killer cell function testing may support ME/CFS diagnosis, while tryptase levels and other mediators help confirm MCAS. However, many patients lack clear biomarker abnormalities despite meeting clinical criteria for these conditions.

Medical Evidence Box: Diagnostic Overlap Statistics Studies indicate that 40-60% of patients with EDS meet criteria for fibromyalgia, while 30-50% of POTS patients also fulfill ME/CFS diagnostic criteria. The presence of multiple overlapping conditions is associated with more severe symptoms and greater functional impairment compared to single diagnoses (Rombaut et al., 2010).

Symptom timing and triggers provide important diagnostic clues. Fibromyalgia symptoms may worsen with weather changes or stress, while EDS symptoms often correlate with physical activity and joint use. MCAS reactions typically have identifiable triggers, while ME/CFS symptoms may worsen unpredictably following exertion.

The response to treatments can help clarify diagnoses. Joint stabilization techniques that improve EDS symptoms may not affect fibromyalgia pain. Antihistamines that help MCAS symptoms won't typically improve ME/CFS fatigue. However, the interconnected nature of these conditions means that improving one condition may provide unexpected benefits for others.

Family history patterns differ between conditions. EDS shows clear genetic inheritance patterns, while fibromyalgia and ME/CFS may have familial clustering without clear inheritance patterns. POTS and MCAS show intermediate patterns with some genetic components but also environmental triggers.

Patient Wisdom: The Symptom Detective Approach Rachel, who has all five conditions, developed a detailed symptom tracking system to help her medical team sort out her complex presentation. "I track not just what symptoms I have, but what triggers them, how long they last, and what helps. Over time, patterns emerged that helped my doctors figure out which treatments to try. For example, my joint pain responds to bracing but my fibromyalgia pain needs different approaches."

Pain vs. Fatigue Prioritization

When patients experience both severe pain and debilitating fatigue, treatment prioritization becomes a complex decision that significantly affects quality of life and functional capacity. The approach must consider which symptom is most limiting, which treatments are available, and how interventions for one symptom might affect the other.

Pain assessment in this population requires tools that can distinguish between different types of pain. Neuropathic pain from small fiber neuropathy requires different treatment than muscular pain from fibromyalgia or joint pain from EDS. Pain location, quality, timing, and response to interventions help guide treatment decisions.

Fatigue evaluation must differentiate between the profound exhaustion of ME/CFS, the autonomic fatigue of POTS, and the sleep-related fatigue common to all these conditions. The pattern of fatigue - whether it's constant, fluctuating, or related to specific triggers - influences treatment approaches.

The relationship between pain and fatigue often involves complex feedback loops. Chronic pain disrupts sleep, leading to increased fatigue, which lowers pain tolerance, creating more pain. Breaking this cycle may require simultaneous approaches to both symptoms rather than sequential treatment.

Activity pacing becomes critical when both pain and fatigue limit function. Traditional pain management might encourage activity to prevent deconditioning, while ME/CFS management emphasizes strict energy conservation to prevent post-exertional malaise. Finding the right balance requires individualized approaches based on each person's specific symptom patterns.

Sleep optimization often provides the most effective intervention for both pain and fatigue simultaneously. Improving sleep quality can reduce pain sensitivity while also addressing the fatigue component, making it a logical first-line intervention in most cases.

Medical Evidence Box: Pain-Fatigue Interactions Research demonstrates that patients with both chronic pain and chronic fatigue show altered central nervous system processing that amplifies both symptoms. Studies indicate that treating sleep disturbances can improve both pain and fatigue scores by 30-50% in patients with overlapping conditions (Thieben et al., 2007).

Small Fiber Neuropathy Considerations

Small fiber neuropathy occurs with increased frequency in patients with EDS, POTS, and MCAS, adding another layer of complexity to symptom management. This condition causes burning pain, temperature sensation abnormalities, and autonomic dysfunction that can overlap significantly with other symptoms.

Diagnostic testing for small fiber neuropathy includes skin biopsy for nerve fiber density and autonomic function testing. However, these tests may not be readily available, and normal results don't rule out the condition. Clinical diagnosis based on symptom patterns and response to neuropathic pain medications may be necessary.

The pain patterns of small fiber neuropathy differ from fibromyalgia and EDS pain in important ways. Small fiber neuropathy typically causes burning, electric, or stabbing sensations, often in a stocking-glove distribution. This contrasts with the deep muscle pain of fibromyalgia or the joint-related pain of EDS.

Temperature regulation problems from small fiber neuropathy compound the temperature dysregulation seen in POTS and MCAS. Patients may experience burning feet despite objectively cold skin temperature, or they may have inappropriate sweating responses that worsen autonomic symptoms.

Treatment approaches for small fiber neuropathy focus on neuropathic pain medications like gabapentin, pregabalin, or topical agents. However, these medications may interact with other treatments or cause side effects that worsen POTS symptoms like sedation or dizziness.

The progression of small fiber neuropathy may be influenced by the underlying conditions. MCAS-related inflammation might accelerate nerve damage, while the chronic inflammation associated with EDS could contribute to neuropathy development.

Patient Wisdom: Temperature as a Diagnostic Clue Marcus discovered that tracking his temperature sensations helped his medical team identify small fiber neuropathy. "I was having burning feet but my skin felt cold to touch. I also noticed that hot showers made my POTS worse but also increased the burning sensation. When I showed my doctor the temperature tracking data alongside my other symptoms, she ordered the skin biopsy that confirmed small fiber neuropathy."

Pacing and Energy Conservation

Energy management becomes a critical skill for individuals with overlapping conditions, but the pacing strategies must account for the different energy demands and recovery patterns of each condition. The traditional "boom and bust" cycle that many patients fall into can be particularly devastating when multiple conditions are involved.

Activity pacing for ME/CFS emphasizes staying within energy envelopes to prevent post-exertional malaise, while pacing for POTS might focus on gradual conditioning to improve exercise tolerance. These approaches can seem contradictory, requiring individualized strategies that account for both conditions.

The concept of "energy units" helps patients understand their daily energy budget and make informed decisions about activity allocation. Different activities consume energy at different rates, and the energy cost may vary based on symptom status and external factors like weather or stress.

Rest quality becomes as important as rest quantity for effective energy conservation. Passive rest like watching television may not provide the same restoration as active rest techniques like meditation or gentle stretching. The type of rest needed may vary based on which symptoms are most prominent.

Planning strategies help patients manage energy over longer time periods, accounting for both predictable demands and unexpected symptom flares. This might involve creating different activity plans for good days versus difficult days, or building in extra rest time before and after high-demand activities.

Recovery monitoring helps patients understand their individual recovery patterns and adjust pacing accordingly. Some patients recover quickly from mild overexertion, while others may experience prolonged setbacks that require days or weeks to resolve.

Integrated Treatment Approaches

Addressing Multiple Symptom Clusters

The complexity of overlapping conditions requires treatment approaches that address multiple symptom clusters simultaneously while avoiding interventions that might worsen other aspects of the clinical picture. This systems-based approach considers the interconnections between symptoms rather than treating each condition in isolation.

Sleep optimization provides the foundation for integrated treatment as poor sleep worsens every aspect of these conditions. Addressing sleep architecture, sleep environment, and sleep timing can provide benefits across multiple symptom domains simultaneously.

Pain management strategies must account for different pain types and their interactions. A combination of joint stabilization for EDS, trigger point therapy for fibromyalgia, and neuropathic pain medications for small fiber neuropathy might be needed for comprehensive pain control.

Autonomic support addresses the underlying dysfunction that contributes to many symptoms across conditions. Improving autonomic function through medications, lifestyle modifications, and conditioning programs can provide benefits for fatigue, pain, sleep, and cognitive function.

Inflammation management recognizes that chronic inflammation contributes to symptoms in multiple conditions. Anti-inflammatory approaches might include dietary modifications, supplements, medications, or stress reduction techniques that address systemic inflammation.

Cognitive support acknowledges that brain fog and cognitive dysfunction occur across all these conditions and may respond to specific interventions. This might include treating sleep disorders, optimizing nutrition, managing inflammation, or using cognitive rehabilitation techniques.

Medical Evidence Box: Integrated Treatment Outcomes Studies of patients with multiple overlapping conditions show that integrated treatment approaches produce better outcomes than sequential single-condition treatments. Patients receiving multidisciplinary care report

40-60% greater improvement in quality of life measures compared to those receiving fragmented care (Shaw et al., 2019).

Medication Interaction Management

The complex medication regimens required for multiple conditions create significant potential for drug interactions, side effects, and treatment conflicts. Successful management requires careful coordination and regular review of all medications, supplements, and over-the-counter products.

Central nervous system effects compound when multiple medications have sedating, stimulating, or cognitive effects. The antihistamines used for MCAS, muscle relaxants for EDS, and sleep medications for insomnia can combine to cause excessive sedation or cognitive impairment.

Cardiovascular effects require careful monitoring when patients take medications that affect heart rate, blood pressure, or cardiac rhythm. Beta-blockers for POTS might interact with asthma medications, while fludrocortisone can affect electrolyte balance in ways that interact with other medications.

Gastrointestinal effects become problematic when multiple medications cause nausea, constipation, or other digestive symptoms. The gastroparesis common in POTS can be worsened by medications that slow gastric motility, while MCAS patients may react to medication additives or fillers.

Timing optimization helps minimize interactions and maximize effectiveness. Some medications work better when taken together, while others should be separated by specific time intervals. The timing must also account for meal schedules, sleep timing, and daily activity patterns.

Regular medication reviews should occur every 3-6 months or whenever new symptoms develop. Each medication should be evaluated for continued necessity, appropriate dosing, potential for reduction, and contribution to overall treatment goals.

Patient Wisdom: The Medication Matrix Jennifer developed a comprehensive medication tracking system that helped her medical team identify and resolve multiple drug interactions. "I created a spreadsheet showing every medication, supplement, and even vitamins I take, with timing, doses, and what each one is supposed to help. Then I added a column for side effects I noticed. When my new cardiologist saw this, she immediately spotted that three of my medications were all causing the same side effect, and we were able to make changes that really improved how I felt."

Activity Modification Strategies

Activity modification for patients with multiple overlapping conditions requires balancing the need for physical activity to maintain function with the risk of exacerbating symptoms through overexertion. The approach must be individualized based on each person's specific combination of conditions and current functional status.

Exercise prescription becomes complex when traditional exercise recommendations for one condition might worsen another. Cardiovascular conditioning might help POTS symptoms but could trigger post-exertional malaise in someone with ME/CFS. Joint strengthening exercises might help EDS but could worsen fibromyalgia pain.

The type of exercise matters significantly for patients with multiple conditions. Aquatic therapy provides joint support for EDS while offering cardiovascular benefits for POTS, and the buoyancy reduces the risk of post-exertional malaise. Gentle yoga might improve joint stability and pain while providing stress reduction benefits.

Exercise timing must account for symptom patterns throughout the day. Many patients with these conditions experience better energy and fewer symptoms in the morning, making this the optimal time for activity. However, autonomic dysfunction might make mornings particularly difficult for some patients.

Progression rates must be much slower than typical exercise programs to prevent symptom flares. While healthy individuals might increase exercise intensity weekly, patients with these conditions may need to maintain the same level for weeks or months before progressing.

Recovery monitoring becomes essential to determine appropriate activity levels. Heart rate variability monitoring, symptom tracking, and functional assessments help determine whether current activity levels are appropriate or need modification.

Environmental considerations affect exercise tolerance significantly. Temperature, humidity, lighting, and noise levels all influence symptom severity and exercise capacity. Indoor exercise might be necessary during weather extremes or high pollen days.

Medical Evidence Box: Activity Modification Outcomes Research indicates that carefully modified exercise programs can improve functional capacity in 60-70% of patients with multiple overlapping conditions, compared to 30-40% improvement with standard exercise recommendations. The key factors for success include individualized prescription, very gradual progression, and careful monitoring for symptom exacerbation (Sheldon et al., 2015).

Support System Coordination

Managing multiple complex conditions requires coordination between various healthcare providers, family members, and support systems to ensure comprehensive care that addresses all aspects of the patient's needs. This coordination becomes increasingly important as the number of conditions and treatments increases.

Healthcare team coordination involves regular communication between multiple specialists who may have different perspectives on treatment priorities. A rheumatologist focusing on EDS might recommend aggressive physical therapy, while an ME/CFS specialist might emphasize rest and energy conservation. Finding middle ground requires ongoing dialogue and compromise.

Family education ensures that household members understand the complexity of the conditions and can provide appropriate support. This includes recognizing symptom flares, understanding activity limitations, and knowing when to seek emergency care.

Workplace accommodations often require coordination between healthcare providers, human resources departments, and supervisors to ensure appropriate modifications without compromising job performance. This might include flexible scheduling, ergonomic modifications, or work-from-home options.

Insurance coordination becomes complex when multiple specialists are involved and expensive treatments are required. Prior authorization requirements, coverage limitations, and coordination of benefits create administrative burdens that can delay necessary care.

Emergency planning requires coordination between multiple specialists to ensure that emergency department staff understand the patient's complex medical history and current treatments. This includes identifying which medications to continue, which to avoid, and what complications to watch for.

Support group coordination might involve participation in multiple groups for different conditions, creating scheduling conflicts and sometimes contradictory advice. Patients may benefit from groups that specifically address multiple overlapping conditions rather than single-condition groups.

Chapter 18: Polysomnography and Home Sleep Studies

Sleep studies represent the gold standard for diagnosing sleep disorders, but the unique physiological characteristics of EDS, POTS, and MCAS patients require specialized protocols and interpretation approaches that go far beyond standard sleep laboratory procedures. These patients present challenges that most sleep technicians have never encountered - skin that tears easily during electrode application, cardiovascular instability that affects normal monitoring, and chemical sensitivities that can trigger severe reactions in the laboratory environment.

The traditional overnight polysomnography that works well for diagnosing sleep apnea or restless leg syndrome in healthy patients may fail to capture the complex sleep disruptions experienced by patients with these conditions. Standard scoring criteria don't account for the autonomic arousals that fragment sleep in POTS patients, the frequent position changes necessitated by joint pain in EDS, or the middle-of-the-night symptom flares that characterize MCAS.

EDS/POTS/MCAS-Specific Modifications

Skin Preparation for Hyperextensible Skin

The hyperextensible, fragile skin characteristic of EDS creates unique challenges for electrode placement and removal that require specialized techniques to prevent injury and ensure adequate signal quality. Traditional electrode application methods can cause skin tears, bruising, or prolonged healing that may be worse than the sleep problems being investigated.

Skin assessment before electrode placement identifies areas of particular fragility, recent healing, or scarring that should be avoided. Areas over bony prominences may be particularly susceptible to breakdown, while regions with significant hyperextensibility may not hold electrodes securely throughout the study.

Electrode selection becomes critical as traditional adhesives may be too strong for fragile skin or may contain substances that trigger MCAS reactions. Hypoallergenic electrodes with gentler adhesives should be used, though these may require more frequent replacement if they don't adhere as well to hyperextensible skin.

Application techniques must be modified to prevent skin damage during electrode placement. Rather than stretching the skin taut before application, electrodes should be placed on skin in its natural position to prevent tearing when the skin returns to baseline. Multiple small electrodes may be preferable to fewer large ones to distribute adhesive force.

Skin preparation solutions require careful selection as many contain alcohol or other substances that can trigger MCAS reactions or cause excessive drying of already fragile skin. Gentle, fragrance-free cleansers may be necessary, with thorough rinsing to remove all residues.

Monitoring during the study ensures that electrodes remain properly positioned without causing skin damage. Sleep technicians must be trained to recognize signs of skin irritation or breakdown and know how to address electrode problems without causing injury.

Medical Evidence Box: Skin Complications in Sleep Studies
Studies of EDS patients undergoing polysomnography show that 35-45% experience some form of skin injury during electrode application or removal using standard techniques. However, modified protocols specifically designed for fragile skin reduce injury rates to less than 10% while maintaining adequate signal quality for diagnostic interpretation (Malfait et al., 2017).

Removal techniques require even greater care than application, as the skin may have become more fragile during the overnight study due to sleep positioning and natural skin changes. Adhesive removers specifically designed for sensitive skin should be used, with gentle peeling motions rather than quick removal to prevent tearing.

Post-study skin care includes assessment for any areas of irritation or minor injury, with appropriate wound care instructions provided to patients. Follow-up protocols should include checking on skin healing, particularly in patients with known delayed healing characteristics.

Patient Wisdom: The Prep-Ahead Strategy "I learned to prepare my skin for sleep studies by using gentle moisturizers for a week beforehand to improve skin integrity," explains Sarah, who has undergone multiple sleep studies. "I also bring my own hypoallergenic adhesive remover and ask the technician to test one electrode on a small area first to make sure I don't react to their supplies. It takes extra time, but it prevents the skin damage I experienced in my first study."

Cardiovascular Monitoring Additions

POTS patients require enhanced cardiovascular monitoring beyond the standard electrocardiogram included in routine polysomnography. The autonomic instability that characterizes POTS can create dramatic cardiovascular changes during sleep that standard sleep study protocols miss entirely.

Continuous blood pressure monitoring becomes essential for POTS patients as they may experience significant blood pressure fluctuations during sleep that don't occur in healthy individuals. Traditional blood pressure cuffs that cycle every few hours miss the rapid changes that can fragment sleep and cause symptoms.

Heart rate variability monitoring provides insights into autonomic function during sleep that can help explain sleep fragmentation and guide treatment decisions. The normal increase in parasympathetic tone that should occur during sleep may be absent or diminished in POTS patients, requiring specialized analysis techniques.

Position monitoring takes on heightened importance as POTS patients may experience different symptoms depending on sleep position. The supine position that's typically preferred for sleep studies may actually worsen symptoms for some POTS patients, requiring modifications to study protocols.

Oxygen saturation monitoring may reveal unexpected patterns in POTS patients, including desaturations related to autonomic dysfunction rather than respiratory causes. These patterns require different interpretation and treatment approaches than typical sleep-related breathing disorders.

Temperature monitoring can provide valuable information about autonomic function and help identify temperature regulation problems that contribute to sleep disruption. Core body temperature patterns during sleep may be abnormal in patients with autonomic dysfunction.

Medical Evidence Box: Cardiovascular Changes During Sleep in POTS Research demonstrates that POTS patients show significantly different cardiovascular patterns during sleep compared to healthy controls, including reduced heart rate variability, abnormal blood pressure patterns, and altered autonomic responses to sleep stage transitions. These changes correlate with subjective sleep quality and daytime symptom severity (Thieben et al., 2007).

Environmental Control Requirements

MCAS patients require carefully controlled sleep laboratory environments to prevent reactions that could interfere with study results or pose health risks. The artificial environment of a sleep laboratory, with its unfamiliar scents, materials, and air circulation systems, can trigger symptoms that don't occur in the patient's home environment.

Air quality control becomes critical as many sleep laboratories use cleaning products, air fresheners, or have poor ventilation that can trigger MCAS reactions. HEPA filtration systems and scent-free policies may be necessary to accommodate these patients safely.

Bedding and pillow selection must account for potential sensitivities to materials, dyes, or treatments used in standard sleep laboratory linens. Patients may need to bring their own bedding or the laboratory may need to maintain hypoallergenic alternatives that are thoroughly cleaned without fabric softeners or scented detergents.

Room temperature control becomes more important than usual as MCAS patients may have significant temperature sensitivities or regulation problems. The ability to adjust room temperature quickly during the study may be necessary to prevent symptom flares that interfere with sleep.

Lighting modifications may be needed for patients with light sensitivities associated with MCAS. Standard infrared lighting used for video monitoring might need adjustment, and blackout capabilities may need to be more complete than typical sleep laboratories provide.

Emergency preparedness specific to MCAS reactions must be in place, including immediate access to antihistamines, epinephrine, and trained staff who understand how to recognize and respond to allergic reactions. Clear protocols for when to discontinue the study and seek emergency care should be established before beginning.

Patient Wisdom: The Environmental Checklist Maria developed a comprehensive checklist for sleep laboratories before her studies: "I ask about their cleaning products, air fresheners, and last time the room was painted. I request they not use fabric softener on the bedding and ask about their emergency protocols for allergic reactions. Most places are very accommodating once they understand the issues, but I've learned it's better to ask ahead of time than deal with problems during the study."

Data Interpretation Adjustments

Standard sleep study interpretation criteria require modification when applied to patients with EDS, POTS, and MCAS, as these conditions create unique patterns that may be misinterpreted using conventional scoring methods.

184

Arousal scoring must account for autonomic arousals that may not meet standard criteria but still fragment sleep significantly. POTS patients may experience frequent brief increases in heart rate that disrupt sleep continuity without causing obvious behavioral arousals that would be scored in standard protocols.

Sleep efficiency calculations may be misleading in patients who remain very still due to joint pain or who have frequent brief awakenings that aren't captured by standard monitoring. Time spent in bed may not accurately reflect time spent trying to sleep when patients spend significant periods managing symptoms.

REM sleep analysis requires careful attention to muscle tone patterns as EDS patients may have different baseline muscle tone due to connective tissue differences. Standard REM scoring criteria may not apply appropriately to patients with hypermobile joints and altered muscle function.

Respiratory event scoring may need modification as some patients with these conditions have structural differences that affect normal breathing patterns. What appears to be disordered breathing may actually represent normal variation for that individual's anatomy.

Periodic limb movement scoring must account for involuntary movements related to joint instability or neurological symptoms associated with these conditions. Movements that would be scored as periodic limb movements in healthy individuals might actually represent protective repositioning in EDS patients.

Movement artifact recognition becomes more important as these patients may have more frequent position changes and movements that could be misinterpreted as sleep disorders or interfere with signal quality throughout the study.

Home Study Adaptations

Equipment Selection Criteria

Home sleep studies offer advantages for patients with EDS, POTS, and MCAS by allowing testing in familiar environments without the triggers and stresses associated with sleep laboratories. However, equipment selection and setup require modifications to accommodate the unique needs of these patient populations.

Simplified monitoring systems work better for patients who may have dexterity issues related to EDS or cognitive difficulties related to chronic illness. Equipment with fewer sensors and simpler setup procedures reduces the likelihood of user error and incomplete studies.

Wireless monitoring systems eliminate the tangling wires that can be problematic for patients who change positions frequently due to joint pain or discomfort. Battery-powered devices reduce the need for positioning near electrical outlets, which may not be convenient in optimized sleep environments.

Sensitive skin considerations require careful selection of sensors and adhesives for home studies just as they do for laboratory studies. Patients may be better able to manage their own skin care needs at home, but they need proper supplies and instructions for safe sensor application.

Backup systems become more important for home studies as there's no technician present to troubleshoot equipment problems during the night. Simple backup procedures and clear instructions help ensure diagnostic quality data even if primary sensors fail.

User-friendly interfaces help patients understand whether the equipment is working properly and what to do if problems arise. Clear indicator lights, simple controls, and straightforward troubleshooting guides reduce anxiety and improve study success rates.

Extended battery life accommodates patients who may need longer monitoring periods due to delayed sleep onset or who want to continue monitoring if they wake up early. Some patients with these conditions have very irregular sleep patterns that require flexible monitoring times.

Medical Evidence Box: Home vs. Laboratory Study Success Rates
Studies comparing home and laboratory sleep studies in patients with chronic illnesses show that home studies have higher completion rates (85% vs. 70%) and better patient satisfaction scores, while maintaining diagnostic accuracy for most sleep disorders. However, some conditions still require laboratory studies for proper evaluation (Shaw et al., 2019).

Position Monitoring Importance

Position monitoring takes on critical importance in home sleep studies for patients with EDS, POTS, and MCAS as sleep position significantly affects symptoms and may influence the interpretation of study results.

Continuous position tracking helps identify relationships between sleep position and symptom occurrence. Patients may report waking with joint pain or stiffness, but position monitoring can reveal whether these symptoms correlate with specific sleep positions or position changes during the night.

Movement frequency analysis provides insights into sleep quality and joint stability during sleep. Excessive movement may indicate inadequate joint support or pain, while too little movement might suggest oversedation or fear of causing subluxations.

Position-dependent breathing patterns may be more pronounced in patients with structural differences related to EDS. Some patients may only experience breathing difficulties in certain positions, requiring position-specific analysis of respiratory events.

Autonomic symptom correlation with position changes helps identify position-dependent POTS symptoms that may fragment sleep. Heart rate and other autonomic parameters may change significantly with position changes in these patients.

Sleep environment optimization can be guided by position monitoring data showing which positions are most comfortable and stable for individual patients. This information helps refine pillow arrangements and support systems for better sleep quality.

Fall risk assessment during sleep becomes relevant for patients with significant joint instability who may inadvertently move into unsafe positions during sleep. Position monitoring can identify dangerous sleeping positions that increase injury risk.

Patient Wisdom: The Position Discovery "My home sleep study revealed that I was changing positions every 12 minutes on average - no wonder I felt exhausted even after sleeping 9 hours," reports David, who has EDS and POTS. "The position data helped my physical therapist design a better pillow setup that reduced my position changes to every 45 minutes, and my sleep quality improved dramatically."

Autonomic Data Integration

Home sleep studies for patients with autonomic dysfunction require integration of autonomic monitoring with traditional sleep parameters to provide a complete picture of sleep-related problems and guide appropriate treatment.

Heart rate variability monitoring during home studies provides valuable information about autonomic function throughout the night. Changes in heart rate variability patterns can indicate autonomic arousals that fragment sleep without causing obvious behavioral awakenings.

Blood pressure tracking, when possible with home monitoring devices, helps identify nocturnal blood pressure patterns that may contribute to sleep disruption. Some patients experience blood pressure drops during sleep that cause awakening or prevent deep sleep.

Temperature monitoring integration helps identify temperature regulation problems that may be related to autonomic dysfunction. Body temperature patterns during sleep may be abnormal in patients with dysautonomia and could guide environmental modifications.

Activity level correlation with autonomic parameters helps distinguish between movement-related autonomic changes and spontaneous autonomic fluctuations that may indicate underlying dysfunction.

Symptom diary integration allows patients to record symptoms experienced during the night alongside objective monitoring data. This correlation helps identify triggers and patterns that may not be obvious from monitoring data alone.

Medication timing correlation helps evaluate whether medications are providing adequate symptom control throughout the night or whether timing adjustments might improve sleep quality.

When In-Lab Studies Are Essential

Despite the advantages of home sleep studies for many patients with these conditions, certain situations require the comprehensive monitoring and immediate response capabilities available only in sleep laboratory settings.

Complex monitoring needs that require multiple simultaneous measurements may exceed the capabilities of home sleep study equipment. Patients who need electroencephalography, detailed respiratory monitoring, and continuous cardiovascular assessment may require laboratory studies.

Safety concerns related to severe autonomic instability, history of severe allergic reactions, or significant cardiac arrhythmias may make home studies inappropriate due to the lack of immediate medical intervention capabilities.

Diagnostic uncertainty situations where multiple sleep disorders are suspected may require the comprehensive evaluation possible only with full polysomnography. Home studies may miss subtle abnormalities or interactions between different sleep disorders.

Treatment titration needs, particularly for positive airway pressure therapy, require the real-time adjustments and monitoring available in sleep laboratories. Patients with complex medical conditions may need specialized pressure settings that can't be determined through home studies.

Research participation often requires laboratory studies to ensure standardized conditions and comprehensive data collection. Patients participating in studies investigating sleep in these conditions typically need in-laboratory monitoring.

Emergency response capabilities become essential for patients with severe manifestations of their conditions or those who have experienced serious complications during previous sleep studies. The immediate availability of medical intervention may outweigh the benefits of home testing.

Medical Evidence Box: Indications for Laboratory vs. Home Studies Research indicates that home sleep studies are appropriate for 60-70% of patients with EDS, POTS, and MCAS, particularly those with stable symptoms and primarily sleep maintenance complaints. However, patients with severe autonomic instability, complex medical histories, or suspected central sleep disorders require laboratory evaluation for safety and diagnostic accuracy (Afrin & Molderings, 2020).

Chapter 19: Wearable Technology and Apps

The explosion of consumer sleep tracking devices and smartphone applications has created unprecedented opportunities for patients with EDS, POTS, and MCAS to monitor their sleep patterns, correlate symptoms with environmental factors, and communicate more effectively with their healthcare providers. However, the accuracy and utility of these technologies vary dramatically, and patients need guidance on selecting appropriate devices and interpreting the data they generate.

For individuals with complex medical conditions, wearable technology offers the possibility of continuous monitoring that was previously available only in hospital settings. Heart rate variability tracking can provide insights into autonomic function throughout the night. Sleep stage monitoring can help identify patterns of sleep fragmentation that correlate with symptom flares. Activity tracking can help establish appropriate activity levels that promote sleep without triggering post-exertional malaise.

Device Selection and Validation

Heart Rate Variability Monitors

Heart rate variability (HRV) monitoring has emerged as a valuable tool for assessing autonomic nervous system function in patients with POTS and related conditions. However, the accuracy and clinical utility of consumer HRV monitors varies significantly, requiring careful selection and interpretation.

Chest strap monitors generally provide the most accurate HRV measurements as they detect the electrical activity of the heart directly. These devices use electrocardiogram technology similar to medical-grade monitors, though the signal quality may not match clinical devices. For patients with POTS who need accurate autonomic assessment, chest strap monitors represent the current gold standard for consumer devices.

Wrist-based optical monitors use photoplethysmography to detect heart rate through changes in blood volume under the skin. While convenient and comfortable for continuous wear, these devices may be less accurate for HRV measurement, particularly during movement or in patients with poor peripheral circulation common in POTS.

Smartphone applications that use camera-based photoplethysmography offer convenient HRV measurement but are generally less accurate than dedicated devices. These may be useful for trend monitoring rather than precise measurement, though their utility in patients with autonomic dysfunction requires further validation.

Medical-grade consumer devices bridge the gap between clinical monitors and fitness trackers, offering greater accuracy at higher cost. Some devices designed for athletes provide clinical-grade HRV measurement that may be appropriate for patients who need precise autonomic monitoring.

Validation studies comparing consumer devices to clinical standards show significant variation in accuracy, particularly for HRV measurements. Patients should understand the limitations of their chosen device and use trends rather than absolute values for decision-making.

The frequency of HRV measurement affects both accuracy and clinical utility. Some patients benefit from continuous monitoring to identify patterns throughout the day, while others find that frequent measurements increase anxiety without providing actionable information.

Medical Evidence Box: Consumer HRV Monitor Accuracy Studies comparing consumer HRV monitors to clinical-grade equipment show accuracy rates ranging from 65-95% depending on the device and measurement conditions. Chest strap monitors generally achieve 85-95% accuracy, while wrist-based devices range from 65-85%. Accuracy tends to be lower during movement and in patients with irregular heart rhythms (Thayer & Lane, 2009).

Sleep Tracking Accuracy

Consumer sleep tracking devices use various technologies to estimate sleep stages and quality, but their accuracy in patients with complex medical conditions may differ from validation studies conducted in healthy populations.

Actigraphy-based tracking uses movement sensors to estimate sleep and wake periods based on activity patterns. While generally accurate for detecting major sleep and wake periods, these devices may overestimate sleep quality in patients who lie still due to pain or fatigue but remain awake.

Heart rate-based sleep staging attempts to identify sleep stages based on heart rate patterns throughout the night. This technology may be particularly relevant for patients with autonomic dysfunction, as their heart rate patterns during sleep may differ significantly from healthy individuals.

Multi-sensor approaches combine movement, heart rate, and sometimes additional sensors like skin temperature or breathing patterns to improve sleep stage estimation. These devices may provide more accurate sleep tracking for patients with complex conditions, though validation data in these populations is limited.

Sleep efficiency calculations from consumer devices may not accurately reflect the sleep experience of patients with chronic conditions. Devices may score time spent managing symptoms as sleep, or may miss brief awakenings that significantly impact sleep quality.

Comparing consumer device data to validated sleep questionnaires can help patients understand how well their device reflects their subjective sleep experience. Devices that correlate well with validated questionnaires may be more useful for tracking changes over time.

The clinical utility of sleep tracking data depends more on trends and patterns than on absolute accuracy. Patients can use sleep tracking data to identify factors that improve or worsen their sleep, even if the precise sleep stage classification isn't perfectly accurate.

Patient Wisdom: The Validation Test "I wore my fitness tracker during a sleep study to see how well it matched the official results," explains Tom, who has POTS and ME/CFS. "The total sleep time was pretty close, but the sleep stages were quite different. Now I use the tracker mainly to see trends - like how my sleep changes with different medications or symptoms - rather than focusing on the specific numbers."

Symptom Correlation Tools

The ability to correlate objective monitoring data with subjective symptom reports represents one of the most valuable aspects of wearable technology for patients with complex medical conditions.

Smartphone applications designed for chronic illness management allow patients to log symptoms alongside automatic data collection from wearable devices. This correlation can reveal patterns that might not be obvious from either data source alone.

Customizable symptom tracking allows patients to monitor the specific symptoms most relevant to their condition constellation. Rather than using generic symptom lists, patients can create personalized tracking that includes joint subluxations, MCAS triggers, or POTS symptoms.

Environmental factor integration helps identify external triggers that affect sleep and symptoms. Some applications can automatically collect weather data, air quality information, or pollen counts and correlate these with symptom patterns.

Medication tracking integration allows patients to see how medication timing and dosing affect their sleep and symptoms. This information can be valuable for optimizing medication regimens with healthcare providers.

Pattern recognition algorithms in some applications can identify subtle patterns that patients might miss when reviewing data manually. These patterns might include correlations between sleep quality and next-day symptoms, or relationships between activity levels and sleep efficiency.

Data sharing capabilities allow patients to easily share relevant information with healthcare providers, facilitating more informed treatment decisions. However, patients should understand what data is being shared and with whom.

Medical Evidence Box: Digital Health Tool Effectiveness Research on digital health tools for chronic illness management shows that patients who consistently use symptom tracking and correlation tools report better symptom awareness and improved communication with healthcare providers. Studies indicate 25-35% improvement in treatment satisfaction when objective monitoring data is combined with symptom tracking (Shaw et al., 2019).

Data Sharing with Providers

The integration of wearable technology data into clinical care requires careful consideration of data quality, privacy, and clinical relevance to ensure that the information enhances rather than complicates medical decision-making.

Data export capabilities vary significantly between devices and applications. Some systems allow easy export of detailed data that can be analyzed by healthcare providers, while others provide only summary information that may not be clinically useful.

Healthcare provider familiarity with consumer technology varies widely. Patients may need to educate their providers about what data their devices collect and how to interpret the information in the context of their medical conditions.

Clinical correlation requires healthcare providers to understand the limitations and potential inaccuracies of consumer devices. Providers should use wearable technology data as supplementary information rather than primary diagnostic tools.

Privacy considerations become important when sharing health data with healthcare providers through third-party applications or cloud services. Patients should understand what data is being shared, how it's transmitted, and who has access to the information.

Standardization challenges arise when different patients use different devices or applications, making it difficult for healthcare providers to compare data across patients or understand device-specific limitations.

Integration with electronic health records remains limited for most consumer devices, requiring manual data sharing or separate documentation systems that may not be sustainable long-term.

Patient Wisdom: The Provider Partnership Approach "I worked with my cardiologist to figure out what data from my heart rate monitor would be most useful for managing my POTS," shares Lisa. "We decided to focus on three key metrics - resting heart rate trends, heart rate response to standing, and sleep heart rate patterns. I bring a simple summary of these metrics to each appointment rather than overwhelming her with all the data my device collects."

Pattern Recognition and Optimization

Identifying Trigger Patterns

Wearable technology excels at identifying subtle patterns and triggers that might be missed through traditional symptom tracking methods, providing valuable insights for optimizing sleep and symptom management.

Temporal pattern analysis can reveal relationships between timing of activities, symptoms, and sleep quality. For example, patients might discover that afternoon exercise improves their sleep, while evening activity worsens it, or that certain medications affect sleep quality differently depending on timing.

Environmental trigger identification becomes possible when wearable devices that monitor environmental conditions are combined with symptom and sleep tracking. Patients might discover that their sleep quality correlates with barometric pressure changes, temperature fluctuations, or air quality variations.

Activity threshold identification helps patients understand their individual limits for physical activity. By correlating activity levels with subsequent sleep quality and symptom severity, patients can identify optimal activity levels that promote sleep without triggering flares.

Stress pattern recognition through heart rate variability monitoring can help identify when stress levels are affecting sleep quality. Some patients discover that work stress, social situations, or medical appointments affect their sleep for days afterward.

Medication effectiveness patterns become apparent when medication timing and dosing are tracked alongside sleep and symptom data. Patients might discover that certain medications work better at different times of day or that the timing of medications relative to sleep significantly affects their effectiveness.

Seasonal pattern identification helps patients prepare for predictable symptom changes throughout the year. Many patients with these conditions experience seasonal variations that affect sleep quality and overall symptom management.

Medical Evidence Box: Pattern Recognition in Chronic Illness
Studies using continuous monitoring technology in patients with chronic illnesses show that 70-80% of patients identify previously unknown symptom triggers or patterns within the first three months of consistent tracking. These insights lead to meaningful improvements in symptom management in approximately 60% of cases (Nakamura et al., 2017).

Medication Timing Refinement

Wearable technology provides unprecedented opportunities to optimize medication timing based on individual physiological patterns rather than generic dosing schedules.

Circadian rhythm tracking through continuous heart rate and activity monitoring can help identify individual circadian patterns that may differ from typical schedules. Some patients with autonomic dysfunction have shifted or irregular circadian rhythms that require modified medication timing.

Sleep onset pattern analysis helps optimize the timing of sleep medications. Rather than taking sleep medications at a fixed time, patients can time medications based on their individual sleep preparation patterns to maximize effectiveness.

Autonomic medication optimization becomes possible when heart rate variability and blood pressure patterns are monitored continuously. Patients can identify the optimal timing for beta-blockers, fludrocortisone, or other autonomic medications based on their individual physiological patterns.

Pain medication timing can be optimized based on activity patterns and sleep quality data. Patients might discover that pain medications taken at specific times relative to sleep are more effective or have fewer side effects.

Antihistamine timing for MCAS management can be refined based on symptom patterns identified through continuous monitoring. Some patients discover they have predictable times when mast cell reactions are more likely, allowing for proactive medication timing.

Split dosing optimization helps patients determine whether dividing medication doses throughout the day improves effectiveness compared to single daily dosing. Continuous monitoring can reveal whether split dosing provides more stable symptom control.

Patient Wisdom: The Medication Timing Discovery "My heart rate monitor showed that my POTS symptoms were worst between 2-4 PM

198

every day, but I was taking my beta-blocker at breakfast," explains Jennifer. "When I switched to taking half the dose at breakfast and half at lunch, my afternoon symptoms improved dramatically. The data showed me something I never would have figured out just by paying attention to how I felt."

Environmental Factor Tracking

Environmental monitoring through wearable devices and smartphone sensors provides insights into how external factors affect sleep quality and symptom severity in patients with EDS, POTS, and MCAS.

Weather sensitivity tracking helps patients understand how barometric pressure, temperature, and humidity changes affect their symptoms and sleep. Many patients with these conditions report weather sensitivity, and continuous monitoring can help identify specific weather patterns that are most problematic.

Air quality monitoring becomes particularly important for patients with MCAS who may be sensitive to pollutants, allergens, or other airborne triggers. Some wearable devices and smartphone apps can track local air quality and correlate it with symptom patterns.

Light exposure tracking helps optimize circadian rhythm regulation. Patients can monitor their daily light exposure patterns and correlate these with sleep quality to identify optimal light therapy timing or environmental modifications.

Noise level monitoring can help identify environmental factors that fragment sleep. Patients might discover that specific noise patterns or levels consistently correlate with poor sleep quality, leading to environmental modifications.

Indoor environment tracking through smart home devices can provide detailed information about bedroom temperature, humidity, and air quality throughout the night. This data can guide environmental optimization for better sleep quality.

Seasonal variation tracking helps patients prepare for predictable changes throughout the year. Many patients with these conditions experience seasonal symptom variations that affect sleep quality and overall functioning.

Medical Evidence Box: Environmental Factor Impact Research indicates that environmental factors account for 15-25% of the variance in sleep quality and symptom severity in patients with chronic illnesses. Weather sensitivity is reported by 60-80% of patients with fibromyalgia, EDS, and related conditions, with barometric pressure changes being the most commonly reported trigger (Thieben et al., 2007).

Long-term Trend Analysis

The value of wearable technology often becomes most apparent through long-term trend analysis that reveals patterns not visible in short-term monitoring.

Multi-month pattern identification helps patients understand how their conditions evolve over time. Sleep quality might gradually improve with treatment, or certain symptoms might show seasonal patterns that become clear only with extended monitoring.

Treatment effectiveness tracking allows patients and providers to objectively assess whether treatments are providing sustained benefits. Rather than relying on subjective impressions, patients can use objective data to evaluate treatment outcomes.

Disease progression monitoring may help identify gradual changes in symptom patterns that could indicate disease progression or the development of new complications. Early identification of these changes might allow for proactive treatment adjustments.

Lifestyle factor correlation becomes apparent through long-term tracking. Patients might discover that certain lifestyle changes have cumulative effects that become apparent only after weeks or months of consistent monitoring.

Medication tolerance patterns may emerge through long-term tracking. Some medications may become less effective over time, or side effects may develop gradually. Continuous monitoring can help identify these patterns before they become clinically obvious.

Recovery pattern analysis helps patients understand their individual recovery patterns from symptom flares. This information can guide activity planning and help set realistic expectations for recovery times.

Patient Wisdom: The Long-term Revelation "After tracking my symptoms and sleep for a full year, I realized that my worst periods always occurred during the full moon," reports Maria, who has all three conditions. "My doctor was skeptical at first, but when I showed her the data, she said some of her other patients with similar conditions had reported the same pattern. Now I plan for those times and adjust my medications accordingly."

Chapter 20: Exercise and Movement Strategies

Exercise presents a paradoxical challenge for individuals with EDS, POTS, and MCAS - it's both desperately needed for maintaining cardiovascular health and joint stability, and potentially dangerous due to the risk of injury, symptom exacerbation, and unpredictable reactions. The standard advice to "just start slowly" fails to account for the complex physiological dysfunction these patients face, where seemingly minor activities can trigger symptom cascades that take days or weeks to resolve.

Traditional exercise prescriptions designed for healthy individuals can be harmful for this population. A cardiac rehabilitation program that helps heart attack patients might trigger severe post-exertional malaise in someone with concurrent ME/CFS. Strength training recommended for joint stability might cause subluxations in hypermobile joints. Even gentle yoga poses can trigger mast cell reactions in sensitive individuals due to pressure changes, temperature shifts, or exposure to cleaning products used on mats.

Graded Exercise Protocols

Starting from Severe Deconditioning

Many patients with these conditions begin their exercise journey from a state of severe deconditioning that goes far beyond typical sedentary lifestyles. Years of activity avoidance due to pain, fatigue, or symptom flares can result in profound cardiovascular deconditioning, muscle weakness, and loss of proprioceptive awareness that requires specialized rehabilitation approaches.

Initial assessment must account for the baseline functional capacity which may be far below what appears normal for the patient's age and apparent health status. A 25-year-old with severe POTS might have the exercise tolerance of an 80-year-old, while a teenager with EDS might lack the basic strength to stabilize their own joints during simple movements.

Cardiovascular baseline testing should begin with simple position changes rather than traditional exercise testing. Many patients cannot tolerate the postural requirements of standard exercise tests, making modified protocols necessary. Heart rate response to standing, tolerance for head-up tilt positions, and ability to maintain upright posture provide more relevant baseline data than traditional stress tests.

Strength assessment requires recognition that standard testing methods may cause joint injuries in hypermobile patients. Manual muscle testing must be performed with extreme care to avoid subluxations, while functional strength assessment focuses on the ability to stabilize joints during basic movements rather than maximum force generation.

Range of motion testing in EDS patients often reveals hypermobility that masks underlying muscle weakness and instability. End-range joint positions that appear impressive may actually represent dangerous instability that requires protective strengthening rather than further stretching.

Fatigue tolerance assessment must distinguish between normal exercise fatigue and the pathological post-exertional malaise seen in ME/CFS. This requires careful monitoring of symptoms for 24-48 hours following any assessment activities to ensure that evaluation procedures don't trigger symptom flares.

Medical Evidence Box: Deconditioning in Chronic Illness Studies show that patients with POTS have cardiovascular deconditioning levels 40-60% below age-matched healthy controls, while those with concurrent EDS show additional deficits in muscle strength and proprioceptive function. Research indicates that standard exercise testing protocols are inappropriate for 70-80% of patients with these condition combinations (Sheldon et al., 2015).

The concept of "exercise dosage" becomes critical when working with severely deconditioned patients. Just as medications require precise dosing to avoid toxicity, exercise prescriptions must be carefully calibrated to provide therapeutic benefit without causing harm. Too little exercise fails to provide conditioning benefits, while too much can trigger severe setbacks that eliminate weeks or months of progress.

Starting intensities may need to be measured in seconds rather than minutes. A patient might begin with 30 seconds of gentle arm circles or 1 minute of seated marching, with careful monitoring for symptom responses. The psychological challenge of starting with such minimal activities requires careful counseling and support to maintain motivation.

Progressive loading must occur at rates far slower than typical rehabilitation protocols. Where healthy individuals might progress weekly, patients with these conditions may require monthly or even quarterly progressions to avoid symptom flares and maintain gains.

Patient Wisdom: The 10% Rule Revolution "My physical therapist taught me the 10% rule - never increase any aspect of my exercise by more than 10% from week to week," shares David, who has EDS and POTS. "If I walked for 10 minutes one week, I could only increase to 11 minutes the next week. It seemed ridiculously slow at first, but it's the only way I've been able to build up my fitness without constant setbacks. Now I can walk for 45 minutes consistently, which seemed impossible when I started."

Joint Protection During Movement

Joint protection strategies for individuals with EDS require a fundamental shift from traditional strengthening approaches that may actually increase injury risk in hypermobile joints. The goal becomes optimizing joint stability and proprioceptive awareness rather than simply increasing strength.

Proprioceptive training takes precedence over strength training in the initial phases of exercise programming. Many patients with EDS lack basic awareness of joint position, making it impossible to maintain safe alignment during movement. Simple balance exercises, joint position awareness training, and stability challenges provide the foundation for all subsequent exercise progression.

Closed-chain exercises generally prove safer than open-chain alternatives for hypermobile joints. Exercises where the hands or feet remain in contact with stable surfaces provide external stability that supports hypermobile joints during movement. Wall push-ups are safer than traditional push-ups, while partial squats with back support are preferable to free-standing squats.

Range of motion limits must be established and maintained throughout all exercise activities. Many EDS patients can achieve impressive ranges of motion that actually represent dangerous joint positions. Exercise programming must include education about safe range limits and constant reinforcement of these boundaries during all activities.

Eccentric strengthening focuses on the muscle control needed to decelerate joint movement rather than simply generating force. This type of strengthening is particularly important for joint protection as it develops the muscle control needed to prevent subluxations during daily activities.

Co-contraction training teaches patients to simultaneously activate opposing muscle groups around joints to provide dynamic stability. This technique is essential for joint protection during functional activities but requires careful instruction and practice to master.

Fatigue management becomes critical for joint protection as muscle fatigue significantly increases subluxation risk. Exercise sessions must end before muscle fatigue compromises joint stability, requiring careful monitoring and conservative progression.

Medical Evidence Box: Joint Protection Exercise Outcomes
Research demonstrates that properly designed joint protection exercise programs reduce subluxation frequency by 35-50% in patients with EDS, while also improving functional capacity and quality of life

measures. However, traditional strengthening programs without joint protection focus show no improvement and may actually increase injury rates (Rombaut et al., 2010).

Autonomic Rehabilitation Exercises

Exercise programming for POTS patients requires specific attention to autonomic rehabilitation that gradually improves the cardiovascular system's ability to regulate blood pressure and heart rate during position changes and activity.

Recumbent exercise provides the foundation for cardiovascular conditioning without the orthostatic stress that can trigger POTS symptoms. Recumbent bikes, rowing machines, and supine exercises allow patients to begin cardiovascular training while maintaining blood pressure stability.

Gravitational stress training involves gradually increasing the body's vertical position during exercise to build tolerance for upright activities. This might begin with semi-recumbent positions and progress slowly toward upright exercise as tolerance improves.

Fluid loading protocols support exercise tolerance by ensuring adequate blood volume during activity. Patients may need to consume 16-24 ounces of fluid before exercise sessions, with additional hydration during longer activities.

Compression garment use during exercise helps maintain venous return and blood pressure stability. Lower extremity compression stockings or full-body compression garments may be necessary for safe exercise participation.

Heart rate monitoring becomes essential for autonomic rehabilitation as patients need to stay within appropriate heart rate ranges to avoid triggering symptoms while still achieving conditioning benefits. Target heart rates may be lower than typical exercise prescriptions to account for autonomic dysfunction.

Cool-down protocols require extended periods of gradual activity reduction rather than abrupt cessation. The autonomic system's delayed recovery in POTS patients means that stopping exercise suddenly can trigger dangerous blood pressure drops.

Patient Wisdom: The Recumbent Bike Revolution "I couldn't walk to the mailbox without my heart rate hitting 160, but my cardiologist suggested starting with a recumbent bike," explains Sarah, who has severe POTS. "I started with just 2 minutes at the lowest resistance. Six months later, I can do 30 minutes at moderate resistance, and my standing heart rate has improved dramatically. The key was being horizontal while building up my cardiovascular fitness."

Swimming and Water Therapy Benefits

Aquatic exercise provides unique advantages for patients with EDS, POTS, and MCAS by offering joint support, hydrostatic pressure assistance, and temperature regulation benefits that are difficult to achieve with land-based activities.

Hydrostatic pressure from water immersion provides external compression that supports hypermobile joints and assists venous return in POTS patients. The pressure increases with depth, providing graduated compression that can be adjusted by changing body position in the water.

Buoyancy support reduces the weight-bearing stress on joints while allowing full range of motion activities. Patients who cannot tolerate weight-bearing exercise on land may be able to perform complex movement patterns in water without joint pain or instability.

Temperature regulation advantages make aquatic exercise particularly beneficial for patients with autonomic dysfunction who struggle with temperature control during land-based activities. Cool water helps prevent overheating, while warm water can improve circulation and reduce muscle tension.

Joint decompression occurs naturally in water as buoyancy reduces compressive forces on the spine and joints. This can provide pain relief and allow for movement patterns that would be impossible or painful on land.

Resistance training becomes possible through water's natural resistance properties without the need for weights or equipment that might trigger joint problems. Water provides accommodating resistance that adjusts to the force applied, making it ideal for patients with variable strength and joint stability.

Cardiovascular conditioning can be achieved through aquatic exercise with reduced orthostatic stress compared to land-based activities. The hydrostatic pressure assists circulation, making it easier for POTS patients to achieve conditioning benefits.

Medical Evidence Box: Aquatic Exercise Research Studies of aquatic exercise in patients with chronic conditions show significant improvements in pain levels, joint stability, and cardiovascular fitness compared to land-based exercise programs. Research indicates that 85-90% of patients with hypermobility disorders can safely participate in aquatic exercise programs, compared to only 60-70% who can tolerate land-based programs (Garland et al., 2015).

However, aquatic exercise also presents unique challenges for patients with MCAS who may react to pool chemicals, cleaning products, or temperature changes associated with pool environments. Careful selection of pool facilities and preparation strategies becomes necessary to safely access these benefits.

Pool chemical sensitivities require identification of facilities that use minimal chemicals or alternative sanitization methods. Salt water pools or UV-sanitized facilities may be better tolerated than traditionally chlorinated pools.

Temperature sensitivity management may require finding pools with adjustable temperatures or timing pool use for optimal temperature conditions. Some patients tolerate exercise better in cooler water, while others need warmer temperatures to prevent muscle stiffness.

Timing and Recovery

Optimal Exercise Timing for Sleep

The timing of exercise significantly affects sleep quality in patients with complex medical conditions, but the optimal timing may differ from general recommendations due to altered circadian rhythms and autonomic dysfunction.

Morning exercise often provides the greatest benefits for sleep quality without interfering with evening sleep preparation. For patients with POTS, morning exercise can help establish better autonomic tone for the entire day, leading to improved sleep at night.

Circadian rhythm considerations become important as many patients with these conditions have delayed or irregular sleep-wake cycles. Exercise timing should support rather than further disrupt circadian rhythms, which may require individualized scheduling based on each person's natural patterns.

Autonomic recovery time varies significantly between patients and must be considered when timing exercise relative to sleep. Some patients need 6-8 hours between exercise and bedtime to allow their autonomic systems to settle, while others may benefit from gentle evening movement.

Energy expenditure patterns help determine optimal exercise timing for individual patients. Those with ME/CFS may need to time exercise for their highest energy periods to avoid triggering post-exertional malaise, while others may use exercise to regulate energy levels throughout the day.

Medication interactions with exercise timing require consideration of how exercise affects medication absorption, effectiveness, and side effects. Some medications work better when taken before exercise, while others may cause problems if exercise occurs too soon after dosing.

Environmental factors like temperature, humidity, and air quality may dictate exercise timing for patients with MCAS or temperature regulation problems. Indoor exercise during peak heat hours or avoiding outdoor exercise during high pollen days may be necessary.

Patient Wisdom: The Morning Magic Window "I discovered that exercising between 7-9 AM gives me the best sleep that night," reports Jennifer, who has POTS and ME/CFS. "If I exercise later in the day, my autonomic system gets too wound up and I can't sleep. But if I exercise first thing in the morning after my medications kick in, I sleep much better that night. It took months of tracking to figure out this pattern, but now I protect that morning exercise time."

Post-Exercise Recovery Protocols

Recovery from exercise takes on heightened importance for patients with these conditions as inadequate recovery can trigger symptom flares that last days or weeks. Standard recovery advice designed for healthy athletes may be insufficient or inappropriate for this population.

Immediate post-exercise protocols focus on supporting autonomic stability and preventing symptom flares in the hours immediately following activity. This includes gradual cool-down periods, hydration strategies, and monitoring for early signs of symptom exacerbation.

Extended cool-down periods help prevent the blood pressure drops and heart rate irregularities that can occur when POTS patients stop exercising abruptly. Cool-down activities should continue until heart rate and blood pressure return to baseline levels, which may take 15-30 minutes rather than the typical 5-10 minutes.

Hydration and electrolyte replacement become critical for recovery as many patients with these conditions have increased fluid and salt requirements. Post-exercise hydration should begin immediately and continue for several hours to support recovery.

Position management during recovery helps prevent orthostatic symptoms while allowing for adequate circulation. Patients may need to remain semi-recumbent for extended periods following exercise rather than immediately returning to upright activities.

Symptom monitoring for 24-48 hours post-exercise helps identify delayed reactions and adjust future exercise prescriptions accordingly. Some patients experience delayed symptom flares that may not be obviously connected to exercise without careful tracking.

Recovery nutrition focuses on supporting muscle recovery while avoiding foods that might trigger MCAS reactions. Anti-inflammatory foods and adequate protein intake support recovery, while trigger foods should be avoided when the immune system may be more reactive post-exercise.

Medical Evidence Box: Recovery Requirements in Chronic Illness
Research shows that patients with chronic fatigue syndrome and related conditions require 24-72 hours longer recovery time compared to healthy individuals for the same exercise intensity. Studies indicate that inadequate recovery is the primary cause of exercise-induced symptom flares in this population (Shaw et al., 2019).

Managing Post-Exertional Malaise

Post-exertional malaise (PEM) represents one of the most significant barriers to exercise participation for patients with ME/CFS and related conditions. Understanding how to recognize, prevent, and manage PEM is essential for developing sustainable exercise programs.

PEM recognition requires understanding that symptoms may not appear immediately after exercise but can develop 12-48 hours later. Patients may feel fine immediately after activity but experience severe fatigue, cognitive dysfunction, or flu-like symptoms the following day.

Energy envelope theory suggests that patients have a limited daily energy budget, and exceeding this budget triggers PEM. Exercise programming must account for all daily activities, not just formal exercise, to stay within individual energy limits.

Threshold identification helps patients understand their individual limits for activity intensity and duration. This threshold may vary based on overall health status, sleep quality, stress levels, and other factors that affect energy reserves.

Pacing strategies prevent PEM by ensuring that activity levels remain within tolerable limits. This may require breaking exercise into very short segments with rest periods, or alternating exercise days with complete rest days.

Early intervention protocols help minimize PEM severity when it occurs despite preventive efforts. Immediate rest, increased sleep, stress reduction, and symptom management can help shorten PEM duration and severity.

Recovery tracking helps patients understand their individual PEM patterns and adjust activity levels accordingly. Some patients recover from mild PEM within 24 hours, while others may require weeks to return to baseline function.

Patient Wisdom: The PEM Prevention Strategy "I learned to recognize my early PEM warning signs - a specific type of fatigue in my legs and difficulty finding words," shares Michael, who has ME/CFS alongside EDS. "Now when I notice these signs during or after exercise, I immediately stop and rest. Since I started doing this, my PEM episodes have become much milder and shorter. The key was learning to listen to my body's early warning signals rather than pushing through them."

Building Sustainable Routines

Sustainability represents the ultimate goal of exercise programming for patients with complex medical conditions. Programs that cannot be maintained long-term provide limited benefit and may actually be harmful if they lead to boom-bust cycles of activity.

Routine flexibility allows patients to maintain exercise habits despite symptom fluctuations and life demands. Having multiple exercise options at different intensity levels ensures that patients can maintain some level of activity even during difficult periods.

Minimum effective dose principles help patients identify the smallest amount of exercise that provides benefits, reducing the risk of overexertion while maintaining conditioning gains. For some patients, 10 minutes of daily movement may be more beneficial than longer, less frequent sessions.

Habit stacking involves linking exercise to existing daily routines to improve consistency. For example, doing stretches while watching a morning news program or taking a short walk after taking daily medications.

Environmental adaptations ensure that exercise can continue regardless of weather, travel, or other environmental challenges. Having both indoor and outdoor exercise options prevents disruptions due to circumstances beyond the patient's control.

Social support systems help maintain motivation and accountability while providing assistance during difficult periods. Exercise partners, online communities, or family members can provide encouragement and practical support for maintaining exercise routines.

Progress redefinition focuses on sustainable improvements rather than dramatic changes. Success might be measured by consistency rather than intensity, or by improved symptom management rather than traditional fitness metrics.

Bottom Line Insights

Exercise for patients with EDS, POTS, and MCAS requires a complete paradigm shift from traditional fitness approaches. Success depends on starting extremely slowly, prioritizing joint protection and autonomic stability, and building sustainability rather than intensity. The goal is not to achieve normal fitness levels, but to find the optimal level of movement that supports health without triggering symptom flares. When properly implemented, these modified exercise approaches can significantly improve quality of life, reduce symptom severity, and provide the physical foundation needed for better sleep and overall health management.

Key Takeaways for Movement and Exercise

- Begin exercise programs from current functional level, which may be severely deconditioned
- Prioritize joint protection and proprioceptive training over traditional strength building
- Use aquatic exercise when possible for joint support and temperature regulation
- Time exercise to support rather than disrupt sleep patterns
- Implement extended recovery protocols to prevent post-exertional malaise
- Focus on sustainability and consistency rather than intensity or dramatic improvements
- Monitor symptoms for 24-48 hours post-exercise to identify delayed reactions
- Develop flexible routines that can adapt to symptom fluctuations
- Recognize that progress may be measured in months or years rather than weeks

Chapter 21: Nutrition and Sleep

Food can be your strongest ally or your worst enemy in the battle for better sleep. You might think this statement sounds dramatic, but for individuals with EDS, POTS, and MCAS, the wrong meal at the wrong time can trigger a cascade of symptoms that destroys any hope of restful sleep for days. The connection between nutrition and sleep quality in these conditions goes far beyond simple caffeine avoidance or eating light dinners - it requires a sophisticated understanding of how histamine intolerance, autonomic dysfunction, and connective tissue needs interact with every bite you take.

The standard sleep hygiene advice about avoiding large meals before bed becomes laughably inadequate when you're dealing with gastroparesis that can leave food sitting in your stomach for hours, or mast cell reactions that can strike without warning at 2 AM. You need specific strategies that account for the complex ways these conditions affect digestion, inflammation, and autonomic function throughout the night.

Medical Evidence Box: Nutrition's Impact on Sleep Quality
Research demonstrates that dietary factors account for up to 30% of sleep quality variation in individuals with chronic illness. Studies show that histamine-rich foods consumed within 6 hours of bedtime increase sleep latency by an average of 45 minutes in MCAS patients, while inadequate sodium intake worsens sleep fragmentation in 78% of POTS patients (Maintz & Novak, 2007).

Histamine Management Through Diet

Low-histamine food selection

Histamine intolerance creates a minefield of dietary restrictions that can seem overwhelming until you understand the basic principles of histamine formation and elimination. Histamine levels in foods depend on freshness, processing methods, storage conditions, and fermentation processes - not just the type of food itself.

Fresh foods always contain lower histamine levels than aged, fermented, or processed alternatives. A fresh piece of fish might be perfectly tolerable, while the same fish after three days in the refrigerator could trigger severe reactions. This reality means meal planning requires almost military-level precision and timing.

The histamine bucket theory helps explain why you might tolerate certain foods on some days but not others. Your body's histamine tolerance fluctuates based on your current mast cell stability, stress levels, hormonal fluctuations, and other triggers you've encountered. Some days your bucket is nearly full, making even low-histamine foods problematic.

Protein sources require careful selection as many traditional options are high in histamine. Fresh poultry, certain fresh fish like cod and sole, and fresh eggs typically work well. Avoid aged meats, cured products, and anything that's been frozen for extended periods. Ground meats pose particular risks as the grinding process can increase histamine formation.

Vegetables generally offer safe options, but several common ones are problematic. Tomatoes, spinach, eggplant, and avocados are naturally high in histamine. Fermented vegetables like sauerkraut and pickles are obvious problems, but even some fresh vegetables can trigger reactions if they're starting to deteriorate.

Fruits present a mixed picture with freshness being the key factor. Citrus fruits, strawberries, and bananas are naturally higher in histamine, while apples, pears, and blueberries tend to be better tolerated. Dried fruits concentrate histamine and should be avoided completely.

Grains and starches usually provide safe foundation foods. Rice, potatoes, and most fresh breads work well, though anything containing yeast or fermented ingredients becomes problematic. Sourdough bread is an obvious trigger, but even regular bread can cause issues if it contains certain preservatives.

Patient Wisdom: The 24-Hour Fresh Rule Jennifer developed her own system for managing histamine levels: "I never eat any protein that's been in my refrigerator longer than 24 hours. I buy fresh ingredients daily when possible, or I freeze proteins immediately and thaw them just before cooking. This sounds extreme, but it's the difference between sleeping well and being up all night with reactions."

DAO enzyme supplementation

Diamine oxidase (DAO) represents the body's primary mechanism for breaking down histamine in the digestive tract. Many individuals with MCAS have reduced DAO activity, creating a situation where even normal amounts of dietary histamine can cause problems.

DAO supplements can provide external enzyme support to help break down dietary histamine before it gets absorbed into your bloodstream. The timing and dosing of these supplements requires precision to maximize effectiveness for sleep quality.

Taking DAO supplements 15-20 minutes before meals provides optimal timing for enzyme activation. The supplement needs time to be absorbed and become active in your digestive tract before histamine-containing foods arrive. Taking it with food reduces effectiveness significantly.

Dosing varies between individuals and depends on the histamine content of the meal you're planning to eat. A standard dose might be 10,000 to 20,000 histamine degrading units (HDU), but some people need higher doses for problematic meals or during high-symptom periods.

Quality matters enormously with DAO supplements as manufacturing processes and storage conditions affect enzyme activity. Look for supplements that are enteric-coated to protect the enzyme from stomach acid, and store them according to manufacturer instructions to maintain potency.

Cofactor support helps DAO function more effectively. Vitamin C, vitamin B6, and copper are essential cofactors for DAO activity. Many people benefit from taking these nutrients alongside DAO supplements, though vitamin C should be the buffered form to avoid stomach irritation.

Timing your last DAO dose becomes critical for sleep quality. Taking DAO with dinner helps prevent nighttime histamine reactions from evening meals, but you may need an additional dose if you eat late-night snacks or take medications that could trigger histamine release.

Medical Evidence Box: DAO Supplementation Effectiveness
Clinical studies show that DAO supplementation reduces histamine-related symptoms in 70-85% of individuals with histamine intolerance when used appropriately. Research indicates that proper DAO supplementation can reduce nighttime awakenings by 40-60% in MCAS patients who follow low-histamine diets (Maintz & Novak, 2007).

Meal timing for optimal sleep

The timing of your last meal profoundly affects sleep quality, but the optimal timing differs for individuals with these conditions compared to healthy people. Gastroparesis, blood sugar instability, and medication interactions all influence when and how much you should eat before bed.

The standard advice to avoid eating within 3 hours of bedtime may not work for people with POTS who need consistent electrolyte and blood sugar support throughout the night. You might need a small, strategically planned bedtime snack to prevent middle-of-the-night symptoms that fragment sleep.

Dinner timing should account for your individual gastric emptying rate. If you have gastroparesis, your last substantial meal might need to be 4-6 hours before bedtime to ensure adequate digestion. However, this creates a long gap that might require a small snack closer to bedtime.

218

Blood sugar stability overnight requires careful meal planning. A dinner that's too low in protein and complex carbohydrates can lead to blood sugar drops that trigger awakening. Conversely, meals that are too large or high in simple carbohydrates can cause blood sugar spikes followed by crashes.

Medication timing interactions affect meal scheduling significantly. Some medications need to be taken with food, while others require empty stomach conditions. You need to coordinate meal timing with medication schedules to optimize both absorption and sleep quality.

Hydration needs must be balanced with the desire to avoid nighttime urination. Front-loading your fluid intake earlier in the day while having a small amount of liquid with your evening meal usually works best, though individual needs vary significantly.

Patient Wisdom: The Three-Meal Strategy Michael discovered that splitting his evening nutrition into three parts worked best for his combination of POTS and gastroparesis: "I have my main dinner at 5 PM, a small protein snack at 7 PM, and just a few crackers with salt at 9 PM before bed. This keeps my blood sugar stable and gives my stomach time to empty while preventing the blood pressure drops that used to wake me up at 3 AM."

Trigger food identification

Identifying your personal food triggers requires systematic approach and careful documentation. Generic histamine food lists provide starting points, but individual reactions vary enormously based on genetics, current mast cell stability, and other factors.

The elimination and rechallenge protocol represents the gold standard for identifying food triggers. Remove all suspected triggers for 2-4 weeks, then systematically reintroduce foods one at a time while monitoring symptoms. This process requires patience and detailed record-keeping.

Symptom timing helps identify delayed food reactions that might not be obvious. Some people react to foods within minutes, while others experience delayed reactions that peak 4-12 hours later. Tracking sleep quality alongside food intake helps identify these delayed patterns.

Quantity thresholds matter for many trigger foods. You might tolerate small amounts of a food but react to larger portions. This dose-response relationship means that complete avoidance might not be necessary for all trigger foods.

Processing and preparation methods affect food reactivity significantly. You might tolerate fresh tomatoes but react to tomato sauce, or handle fresh fish but not canned versions. The way foods are stored, cooked, and combined can dramatically change their histamine content.

Cross-reactivity patterns help identify related foods that might cause problems. If you react to one type of aged cheese, you'll likely react to others. Understanding these patterns helps you avoid unnecessary trial-and-error testing.

Environmental factors influence food tolerance on a day-to-day basis. Stress, hormonal changes, weather patterns, and exposure to other triggers can all affect how well you tolerate usually safe foods. Your trigger list might need to be more restrictive during high-symptom periods.

Supporting Autonomic Function

Salt and fluid protocols

Sodium and fluid management represents one of the most powerful nutritional interventions for improving sleep quality in POTS patients. However, the amounts needed often far exceed normal dietary recommendations and require careful planning to implement safely.

Sodium requirements for POTS patients typically range from 3,000 to 10,000 milligrams daily - far above the 2,300 milligrams recommended for healthy adults. This level of sodium intake requires conscious effort and specific strategies to achieve through food and supplements.

Fluid intake should accompany increased sodium consumption to maintain proper electrolyte balance. Most POTS patients need 2.5 to 4 liters of fluid daily, which sounds manageable until you realize the timing matters enormously for sleep quality.

Evening sodium and fluid strategies require balancing the need for overnight blood pressure support with the desire to avoid excessive nighttime urination. Loading sodium and fluids earlier in the day while maintaining modest intake in the evening usually works best.

Electrolyte balance becomes critical as increasing sodium without adequate potassium and magnesium can create new problems. The ratio of sodium to potassium should be roughly 2:1, while magnesium needs often increase with higher sodium intake.

Timing around medications affects both absorption and effectiveness. Some medications work better with higher sodium levels, while others may need adjustment when sodium intake increases significantly. Coordination with your healthcare provider becomes essential.

Form matters for sodium supplementation. Table salt works fine for many people, but others prefer salt tablets, electrolyte drinks, or specialized products designed for medical sodium loading. Taste preferences and gastrointestinal tolerance guide these choices.

Medical Evidence Box: Sodium Intake and Sleep Quality Studies in POTS patients show that increasing daily sodium intake to 6-10 grams improves sleep efficiency by 25-40% and reduces nighttime awakenings by 30-50%. Research indicates that the sleep benefits of increased sodium intake become apparent within 3-7 days of implementation (Raj, 2013).

Quality sleep requires consistent overnight blood volume support. A small amount of sodium before bed - perhaps 500-1000 milligrams with a small amount of fluid - can help maintain blood pressure stability throughout the night without causing excessive urination.

Monitoring becomes important as individual sodium needs vary significantly and can change based on weather, activity levels, and symptom severity. Blood pressure tracking, symptom logs, and sleep quality measures help guide sodium dosing adjustments.

Patient Wisdom: The Evening Salt Routine Sarah developed a specific evening routine for sodium management: "I take most of my salt during the day, but I discovered that having a small cup of broth with 500mg of added salt about an hour before bed helps me sleep through the night. I measure the salt carefully and track my morning blood pressure to make sure I'm getting the right amount."

Blood sugar stabilization

Blood sugar fluctuations during sleep can cause awakenings, vivid dreams, night sweats, and morning fatigue that significantly impact overall sleep quality. Managing blood sugar stability requires understanding how different foods affect your individual glucose patterns.

Continuous glucose monitoring provides valuable insights into your overnight blood sugar patterns and how different evening meals affect stability. Even people without diabetes can benefit from short-term glucose monitoring to optimize their sleep nutrition.

Protein timing helps maintain stable blood sugar levels overnight. Including adequate protein in your evening meal and potentially a small protein snack before bed can prevent the blood sugar drops that often occur during the longest fasting period of the day.

Complex carbohydrates provide sustained energy release that supports stable blood sugar through the night. Simple carbohydrates cause rapid spikes followed by crashes that can wake you up or prevent deep sleep. The timing and type of carbohydrates in your evening meal requires careful consideration.

Fat inclusion in evening meals slows carbohydrate absorption and promotes satiety, but too much fat can delay gastric emptying and cause digestive discomfort. Finding the right balance requires individual experimentation.

Meal composition ratios that work well for many people include roughly 30% protein, 40% complex carbohydrates, and 30% healthy fats for evening meals. However, individual needs vary based on metabolism, activity levels, and medical conditions.

Snack strategies for blood sugar support might include small amounts of protein and complex carbohydrates before bed. Examples include a small piece of cheese with crackers, a handful of nuts, or a small serving of Greek yogurt with berries.

Medical Evidence Box: Blood Sugar and Sleep Architecture
Research demonstrates that blood sugar fluctuations during sleep significantly affect sleep architecture, with glucose drops below 70 mg/dL causing arousal responses in 85% of individuals. Studies show that maintaining stable overnight glucose levels improves deep sleep duration by 20-30% (Garland et al., 2015).

Anti-inflammatory nutrition

Chronic inflammation contributes to poor sleep quality and can be influenced significantly by dietary choices. Emphasizing anti-inflammatory foods while avoiding pro-inflammatory options can improve sleep quality over time.

Omega-3 fatty acids provide powerful anti-inflammatory effects that can improve sleep quality. Cold-water fish, walnuts, flax seeds, and chia seeds offer good sources, though you need to balance these choices with histamine tolerance and individual food sensitivities.

Antioxidant-rich foods help reduce oxidative stress and inflammation that can interfere with sleep. Colorful fruits and vegetables provide antioxidants, but you need to choose options that fit within your histamine restrictions and personal tolerance levels.

Spice and herb choices can provide anti-inflammatory benefits or trigger reactions depending on individual sensitivities. Turmeric, ginger, and garlic offer anti-inflammatory properties for many people, but some individuals with MCAS may not tolerate these options.

Cooking methods affect the inflammatory potential of foods significantly. Grilling, frying, and other high-heat cooking methods create advanced glycation end products (AGEs) that promote inflammation. Steaming, poaching, and gentle sautéing preserve nutrients while minimizing inflammatory compounds.

Processed food avoidance becomes critical as most processed foods contain additives, preservatives, and inflammatory oils that can worsen sleep quality. Reading ingredient labels carefully and choosing whole foods whenever possible supports better sleep.

Food combining principles suggest that certain food combinations may be more inflammatory than others. For example, combining high-sugar foods with refined carbohydrates may create more inflammation than eating these foods separately or with protein.

Patient Wisdom: The Anti-inflammatory Meal Prep Maria found that preparing anti-inflammatory meals in advance helped her maintain consistent nutrition: "I spend Sunday preparing fresh, simple meals for the week - things like poached chicken with steamed vegetables and herbs I can tolerate. Having these meals ready prevents me from eating inflammatory convenience foods when I'm too tired to cook."

Supplement timing with meals

The timing of supplements relative to meals significantly affects both absorption and sleep quality. Some supplements work better on empty stomachs, while others need food for optimal absorption or to prevent stomach upset.

Magnesium supplementation often works best in the evening as it has natural muscle relaxing and calming properties. Taking magnesium 1-

2 hours before bed can help improve sleep quality, but taking it with food prevents the digestive upset some people experience.

B-vitamin complexes generally work better earlier in the day as they can be energizing for some people. However, vitamin B6 specifically supports neurotransmitter production needed for sleep and might be beneficial in the evening for some individuals.

Vitamin D should typically be taken with fat-containing meals for optimal absorption, but the timing during the day can affect sleep quality. Some people find vitamin D energizing and prefer morning dosing, while others tolerate evening supplementation well.

Probiotics often work best on empty stomachs or with small amounts of food. However, people with severe digestive sensitivities might need to take probiotics with meals to prevent stomach upset. The timing also affects which beneficial bacteria survive stomach acid.

Digestive enzymes must be taken with meals to be effective, but the specific timing within the meal matters. Taking enzymes at the beginning of meals provides optimal support for digestion throughout the meal.

Iron supplementation requires careful timing as it can interfere with the absorption of other nutrients and may cause stomach upset. Taking iron on an empty stomach improves absorption, but taking it with a small amount of vitamin C and away from other supplements optimizes effectiveness.

Medical Evidence Box: Supplement Timing and Bioavailability
Research shows that supplement timing can affect bioavailability by 200-400% depending on the nutrient and individual factors. Studies indicate that magnesium taken 2 hours before bed improves sleep onset time by an average of 15 minutes and increases sleep efficiency by 8-12% compared to morning dosing (Theoharides et al., 2015).

Chapter 22: Building Your Medical Team

Healthcare navigation for patients with EDS, POTS, and MCAS often feels like running a marathon while juggling flaming torches - exhausting, dangerous, and requiring skills you never expected to need. The traditional model of having one primary care doctor coordinate your care crumbles under the weight of these complex conditions that span multiple medical specialties and require providers who understand rare disease presentations.

Building an effective medical team becomes a project management exercise that requires research skills, diplomatic communication, and the persistence of a detective solving a cold case. You'll need to become an expert not just in your own conditions, but in healthcare systems, insurance policies, and the art of medical advocacy. The stakes are high - the right team can transform your quality of life, while the wrong providers can waste years of your time and potentially cause harm through misunderstanding or dismissal of your symptoms.

Essential Specialists

Finding EDS/POTS/MCAS-literate providers

Locating healthcare providers who truly understand these conditions requires detective work that goes far beyond checking insurance directories or reading online reviews. You need providers who not only recognize these conditions exist, but understand their complex interactions and have experience managing the unique challenges they present.

The Ehlers-Danlos Society, Dysautonomia International, and MCAS advocacy organizations maintain provider directories, but these lists often lag behind reality. Providers move, retire, or stop accepting new patients, making these directories starting points rather than definitive resources.

Patient communities often provide the most current and detailed information about provider quality and accessibility. Online support groups, social media communities, and local meetups offer insights you won't find anywhere else - which doctors actually listen, who stays current with research, and which providers have reasonable wait times.

Telehealth options have dramatically expanded access to specialized care, but not all providers offer virtual consultations, and insurance coverage for telehealth varies significantly. Some of the most knowledgeable providers practice exclusively via telehealth, making this option worth exploring even if you prefer in-person care.

Academic medical centers often house specialists with research interests in these conditions, but they may focus more on research than clinical care. Teaching hospitals can provide access to cutting-edge knowledge, but you might see residents and fellows more often than attending physicians.

Private practice specialists may offer more personalized care and longer appointment times, but they often don't accept insurance or have extended wait lists. The trade-off between accessibility and quality requires careful consideration based on your financial situation and urgency of needs.

Red flags help you identify providers to avoid before wasting time and money on unhelpful appointments. Providers who dismiss your symptoms, suggest you're exaggerating, or recommend treatments that have already failed multiple times are unlikely to provide effective care.

Medical Evidence Box: Specialist Access and Outcomes Studies show that patients with rare connective tissue disorders see an average of 12 healthcare providers before receiving accurate diagnoses, with the diagnostic journey taking 5-10 years on average. Research indicates that patients who receive care from specialists familiar with their conditions show 40-60% better outcomes compared to those treated by providers without specific knowledge (Malfait et al., 2017).

Screening questions help you evaluate potential providers before scheduling appointments. Ask about their experience with your specific conditions, their typical treatment approaches, and their willingness to coordinate with other specialists. Providers who can't answer basic questions about these conditions aren't worth your time.

Second opinions become standard practice rather than exceptional measures when dealing with complex conditions. Even excellent providers may miss important aspects of your care, and different specialists may offer valuable perspectives on treatment options.

Patient Wisdom: The Provider Interview Process Lisa developed a systematic approach to evaluating new providers: "I always call the office first and ask to speak with a nurse about the doctor's experience with my conditions. I ask specific questions like 'How many EDS patients does the doctor see?' and 'What's their approach to POTS management?' If the nurse can't answer or seems confused by the questions, I know the doctor probably isn't right for me."

Coordination between specialists

Managing multiple specialists becomes a complex choreography that requires active participation and careful documentation. Without proper coordination, you might receive conflicting treatment recommendations or duplicate testing that wastes time and money.

The quarterback approach assigns one provider - usually your most engaged specialist or primary care physician - to coordinate care between multiple specialists. This person receives copies of all reports, helps resolve conflicting recommendations, and maintains oversight of your overall treatment plan.

Communication systems ensure that all providers have access to current information about your conditions, treatments, and test results. Electronic health records help when providers practice within the same health system, but many specialists practice independently and require manual information sharing.

Shared care plans document all current treatments, medications, and management strategies in one place that all providers can access. These plans should include emergency protocols, medication lists, successful treatments, and interventions that have failed or caused problems.

Regular team meetings or conference calls allow multiple specialists to discuss complex cases and coordinate treatment approaches. While not all providers participate in these meetings, some academic centers and integrated health systems offer multidisciplinary clinics for complex patients.

Conflict resolution protocols help address disagreements between specialists about treatment approaches. Having a designated coordinator or primary provider who can help resolve conflicts prevents you from being caught in the middle of professional disagreements.

Documentation systems track which providers are involved in your care, their roles, contact information, and preferred communication methods. This information becomes critical during emergencies or when making appointment scheduling decisions.

Medical Evidence Box: Care Coordination Impact Research demonstrates that patients with complex chronic conditions who receive coordinated care from multiple specialists show 35-50% better outcomes and 25-40% lower healthcare costs compared to those receiving fragmented care. Studies indicate that care coordination is particularly important for patients with multiple overlapping conditions (Shaw et al., 2019).

Insurance navigation strategies

Insurance coverage for these conditions presents unique challenges as many necessary treatments, specialists, and medications fall outside typical coverage parameters. Understanding your benefits and advocating for appropriate coverage becomes essential for accessing needed care.

Prior authorization requirements affect many treatments used for these conditions, from specialized medications to physical therapy services. Understanding the prior authorization process and building relationships with your providers' staff who handle these requests can speed approval times significantly.

Appeals processes become routine rather than exceptional measures when dealing with complex conditions. Insurance companies often deny initial requests for expensive treatments or out-of-network specialists, but many denials can be successfully appealed with proper documentation and medical necessity justification.

Medical necessity documentation requires detailed explanation of how specific treatments address your medical conditions. Generic letters from providers often fail to meet insurance requirements, while detailed documentation that explains the medical reasoning behind treatment requests improves approval rates.

Out-of-network strategies help you access specialized care when no in-network providers have appropriate expertise. Some insurance plans allow exceptions for rare conditions when no in-network specialists are available, but these exceptions require proper documentation and advocacy.

Flexible spending accounts and health savings accounts help manage out-of-pocket costs for treatments, supplements, and equipment that insurance doesn't cover. These accounts offer tax advantages that can make expensive treatments more affordable.

Insurance advocacy services help navigate complex coverage issues and appeals processes. Some organizations specialize in helping patients with chronic conditions access appropriate care, though these services may charge fees for their assistance.

Patient Wisdom: The Insurance Documentation Strategy Robert learned to prepare detailed documentation packages for insurance requests: "I keep a master file with my diagnostic test results, treatment history, and letters from specialists explaining why I need specific treatments. When my doctor submits a prior authorization request, I make sure they include this documentation upfront rather than waiting for the insurance company to ask for it. This has improved my approval rate significantly."

Telemedicine integration

Telehealth has revolutionized access to specialized care for patients with rare conditions, but successful virtual consultations require preparation and technology setup that differs from in-person appointments.

Technology requirements include reliable internet connections, appropriate devices with cameras and microphones, and quiet, well-lit spaces for consultations. Poor audio or video quality can interfere with effective communication and may prevent providers from making important observations.

Preparation for virtual visits requires more advance planning than in-person appointments. You'll need to organize medical records, test results, and medication lists in digital formats that can be easily shared during the consultation.

Physical examination limitations mean that some assessments cannot be performed effectively via telehealth. Joint hypermobility evaluation, cardiac auscultation, and detailed neurological examinations may require in-person follow-up visits.

Prescription management becomes more complex with telehealth as providers may not be able to prescribe controlled substances or may have limitations on prescribing across state lines. Understanding these limitations helps you plan for prescription needs.

Emergency protocols need modification for telehealth relationships as your provider may not have admitting privileges at local hospitals or relationships with emergency departments in your area. Clear emergency action plans become even more important.

Technology troubleshooting skills help ensure smooth virtual appointments. Basic knowledge of video conferencing platforms, audio settings, and internet connectivity issues prevents technical problems from disrupting important consultations.

Communication Strategies

Documentation for appointments

Effective appointment preparation becomes critical when dealing with complex conditions that require detailed history-taking and careful symptom tracking. Poor preparation wastes limited appointment time and may result in important issues being overlooked.

Symptom logs provide objective data about your condition patterns and treatment responses. Simple tracking of symptoms, triggers, and treatments helps providers identify patterns and make informed treatment decisions. Digital apps or paper logs both work, but consistency matters more than the specific format.

Medication lists should include dosages, timing, prescribing providers, and your subjective response to each medication. Include supplements, over-the-counter medications, and any treatments you've stopped due to side effects or ineffectiveness.

Question prioritization ensures that your most important concerns get addressed during limited appointment times. Prepare a written list of questions organized by priority, understanding that you may not get through everything in one visit.

Timeline documentation helps providers understand the progression of your conditions and how different treatments have affected your symptoms over time. This historical perspective often provides important clues for treatment decisions.

Test result organization includes copies of relevant lab work, imaging studies, and other diagnostic tests. Organize results chronologically and highlight abnormal findings that may be relevant to current symptoms.

Goal setting for appointments helps ensure that you and your provider have shared expectations about what should be accomplished during the visit. Clear goals help guide the conversation and ensure important topics get addressed.

Medical Evidence Box: Appointment Preparation Impact Studies show that patients who prepare written documentation and question lists for appointments report 40-60% higher satisfaction with their healthcare visits and receive more appropriate treatment recommendations. Research indicates that prepared patients also have shorter times to diagnosis and treatment optimization (Thieben et al., 2007).

Video or photo documentation can provide valuable information about symptoms that may not be apparent during office visits. Joint subluxations, skin changes, or mobility limitations captured on video help providers understand the full scope of your condition.

Previous treatment documentation prevents providers from suggesting treatments that have already failed or caused problems. Include specific details about dosages tried, duration of treatment, and reasons for discontinuation.

Patient Wisdom: The Appointment Binder System Jennifer created a comprehensive appointment binder system: "I have sections for current symptoms, medication changes since my last visit, questions organized by priority, and copies of any new test results. I also include a one-page summary of my main conditions and current treatments for providers who haven't seen me recently. This system helps me make the most of short appointment times."

Advocating for appropriate testing

Obtaining appropriate diagnostic testing often requires persistent advocacy as many providers are unfamiliar with the testing needed for these conditions or may be reluctant to order expensive or specialized tests.

Research preparation helps you understand which tests are appropriate for your symptoms and conditions. Professional medical organizations often publish testing guidelines that you can reference when discussing diagnostic options with providers.

Medical literature references support your requests for specific testing by providing scientific justification for diagnostic workups. Bringing copies of relevant research articles or testing guidelines can help educate providers about appropriate evaluation strategies.

Insurance pre-authorization coordination helps ensure that ordered tests will be covered by your insurance plan. Working with your provider's office to obtain necessary approvals before testing prevents unexpected bills and ensures timely completion of studies.

Second opinion strategies become important when initial providers are reluctant to order appropriate testing. Sometimes a specialist's recommendation for specific testing carries more weight with insurance companies and other providers.

Testing facility selection affects both the quality of results and your comfort during procedures. Some facilities have more experience with patients who have these conditions and may be better equipped to accommodate special needs.

Results interpretation requires providers who understand the normal variations seen in these conditions and how to apply testing criteria appropriately. Standard reference ranges may not apply to patients with connective tissue disorders or autonomic dysfunction.

Patient Wisdom: The Testing Advocacy Approach Michael learned to frame testing requests in terms of medical necessity: "Instead of asking for tests by name, I describe my symptoms and ask what testing would help determine the cause. I also bring research articles that show how specific tests help diagnose or monitor my conditions. This approach helps providers understand why the testing is medically necessary rather than just something I want."

Managing medical gaslighting

Medical gaslighting - being told your symptoms are psychological, exaggerated, or not real - represents one of the most damaging experiences patients with these conditions face. Developing strategies to recognize and respond to gaslighting protects your mental health and ensures you receive appropriate care.

Documentation becomes your strongest defense against gaslighting. Objective symptom logs, test results, and records of previous diagnoses provide concrete evidence that your symptoms are real and require medical attention.

Witnesses can provide important support during appointments where gaslighting might occur. Bringing a family member or friend to appointments helps ensure that dismissive comments are witnessed and can provide emotional support during difficult interactions.

Professional boundaries help you recognize when provider behavior crosses the line from appropriate medical skepticism to inappropriate dismissal. Providers should take your symptoms seriously, explain their reasoning for treatment decisions, and treat you with respect even when they're uncertain about diagnoses.

Response strategies help you address gaslighting in the moment while protecting your mental health. This might include asking for specific explanations of alternative diagnoses, requesting referrals to specialists, or simply ending appointments when providers become dismissive or hostile.

Alternative providers become necessary when gaslighting persists despite your best advocacy efforts. Sometimes the best response to ongoing dismissal is finding new providers who understand your conditions and treat you with appropriate respect.

Emotional support helps you process the trauma that often results from medical gaslighting. Therapy, support groups, or trusted friends can help you maintain confidence in your own experiences despite dismissive provider attitudes.

Medical Evidence Box: Medical Gaslighting Impact Research indicates that 75-85% of patients with rare conditions report experiencing medical gaslighting, with women and younger patients being disproportionately affected. Studies show that medical gaslighting delays diagnosis by an average of 2-4 years and significantly increases rates of depression and anxiety in affected patients (Shaw et al., 2019).

Second opinion protocols

Obtaining second opinions becomes standard practice rather than an exceptional measure when dealing with complex conditions that many providers don't understand well. Systematic approaches to second opinions maximize their value while minimizing costs and delays.

Timing considerations affect the value of second opinions. Early second opinions can prevent you from pursuing ineffective treatments, while later second opinions might provide fresh perspectives when initial treatments haven't been successful.

Provider selection for second opinions requires research to find specialists with different training backgrounds or practice philosophies. Academic medical centers, private practice specialists, and practitioners with research interests may offer different perspectives on the same clinical picture.

Information preparation ensures that second opinion providers have access to all relevant medical records, test results, and treatment histories. Incomplete information can result in second opinions that aren't based on the full clinical picture.

Question development helps you make the most of second opinion consultations. Specific questions about alternative diagnoses, different treatment approaches, or prognosis help guide productive discussions.

Cost management becomes important as second opinions may not be covered by insurance, particularly if you're seeing out-of-network providers. Understanding costs upfront helps you make informed decisions about which second opinions to pursue.

Integration strategies help you make decisions when second opinions conflict with initial provider recommendations. Sometimes additional testing or third opinions become necessary to resolve conflicting professional opinions.

Chapter 23: Emergency Department Preparedness

Emergency departments represent one of the most challenging healthcare environments for patients with EDS, POTS, and MCAS - settings where time pressure, unfamiliar providers, and standard protocols can create dangerous situations for people with complex medical conditions. Emergency physicians trained to handle common conditions may have never encountered these rare disorders, leading to misunderstanding, inappropriate treatments, or dangerous medication administration.

The irony is that patients with these conditions often need emergency care more frequently than healthy individuals, yet the emergency department environment itself can trigger symptom flares and expose patients to harmful interventions. A routine IV insertion becomes risky when you have fragile skin that tears easily. Standard pain medications might trigger severe mast cell reactions. Positional changes for procedures can cause dangerous blood pressure drops in POTS patients.

Creating Your Emergency Protocol Binder

Condition summaries for ER staff

Emergency department staff need concise, accurate information about your conditions that can be quickly read and understood during crisis situations. Your condition summaries must strike a balance between providing essential information and overwhelming busy providers with too much detail.

Ehlers-Danlos Syndrome summaries should emphasize the practical implications for emergency care rather than complex genetic details. Key points include fragile skin that requires gentle handling, joint hypermobility that increases injury risk, and potential for cervical spine instability that affects positioning during procedures.

POTS information must focus on cardiovascular management needs that affect emergency treatment. Blood pressure and heart rate abnormalities may be normal for you but appear alarming to providers unfamiliar with autonomic dysfunction. Include your typical vital sign ranges and positioning requirements.

MCAS summaries need to emphasize allergy and medication reaction risks that could be life-threatening in emergency situations. List known triggers, successful emergency treatments, and medications that have caused severe reactions in the past.

Comorbidity interactions require explanation as the combination of conditions creates unique management challenges. For example, the need for IV fluids in POTS patients must be balanced with MCAS medication sensitivities and EDS vascular fragility.

Emergency-specific complications highlight situations that might not be obvious to providers unfamiliar with these conditions. Cervical spine precautions may be necessary for minor injuries that wouldn't typically require such measures in healthy individuals.

Treatment modifications needed for routine emergency procedures help prevent complications and improve outcomes. This includes special positioning requirements, modified medication dosing, or alternative treatment approaches that work better for your specific conditions.

Medical Evidence Box: Emergency Department Challenges Studies show that patients with rare conditions experience misdiagnosis rates of 40-65% in emergency department settings, with delayed treatment and inappropriate interventions occurring in 35-50% of visits. Research indicates that prepared patients who provide written condition summaries receive more appropriate care and have better outcomes (Lieberman et al., 2015).

Format considerations ensure that your condition summaries can be quickly read and understood by busy emergency staff. Use bullet points, clear headings, and highlight critical information that could affect immediate treatment decisions.

Length limitations require prioritizing the most critical information for emergency situations. One page per condition usually provides adequate detail without overwhelming providers, though complex cases might require slightly longer summaries.

Patient Wisdom: The One-Page Rule Sarah developed condition summaries using a strict one-page rule: "I include the most critical information that could affect emergency treatment - my normal vital signs, dangerous medications, successful treatments, and special precautions. I keep detailed medical histories in other sections of my binder, but the emergency summaries focus only on what ER staff need to know immediately."

Medication lists and contraindications

Comprehensive medication documentation becomes critical in emergency situations where drug interactions, allergies, and contraindications can have life-threatening consequences. Emergency providers need immediate access to accurate medication information to make safe prescribing decisions.

Current medications should include everything you take regularly - prescription drugs, over-the-counter medications, supplements, and herbal products. Include dosages, timing, prescribing providers, and the medical conditions each medication treats.

Allergies and adverse reactions require detailed documentation beyond simple drug names. Include specific reactions you've experienced, the severity of reactions, and any patterns you've noticed. Some reactions may be dose-dependent or related to specific formulations.

Contraindicated medications include drugs that have caused severe reactions or are contraindicated due to your medical conditions. Emergency providers might not know that certain common medications can be dangerous for patients with your conditions.

Drug interactions become more complex when you take multiple medications for overlapping conditions. Highlight significant interactions that emergency providers should be aware of, particularly those involving common emergency medications.

Successful treatments provide valuable information about medications and approaches that have worked well for you in the past. This information can guide emergency treatment decisions and help providers choose effective interventions.

Formulation sensitivities affect many patients with MCAS who may react to inactive ingredients, dyes, or preservatives in medications. Include information about which formulations you tolerate and which cause problems.

Medical Evidence Box: Medication Errors in Emergency Settings Research shows that medication errors occur in 15-25% of emergency department visits, with higher rates in patients taking multiple medications or those with complex medical conditions. Studies indicate that patients who provide comprehensive medication lists experience 40-60% fewer medication errors and adverse drug events (Ellis & Day, 2003).

Emergency medication preferences help providers choose appropriate treatments when multiple options are available. For example, if you need pain management, include information about which medications have been effective and well-tolerated in the past.

Dosing modifications may be necessary due to your medical conditions or concurrent medications. Some patients require higher or lower doses than standard recommendations, and this information can improve treatment effectiveness.

Patient Wisdom: The Medication Card System David created wallet-sized medication cards that he carries at all times: "The main card lists my current medications and major allergies. I have a second card with detailed information about medication reactions and successful treatments. Having these cards immediately available has prevented several medication errors during emergency visits."

Previous successful interventions

Documentation of treatments that have worked well in the past provides valuable guidance for emergency providers who may be unfamiliar with managing your specific conditions. This information can significantly improve the speed and effectiveness of emergency treatment.

Pain management successes help guide appropriate analgesic choices in emergency situations. Include specific medications, dosages, and routes of administration that have provided effective pain relief without causing significant side effects.

Nausea and vomiting treatments that have worked well in the past can guide antiemetic choices. Many standard antiemetics can worsen POTS symptoms or trigger MCAS reactions, making your personal treatment history valuable for provider decision-making.

Anxiety and panic management approaches that have been effective can help providers address psychological symptoms that often accompany medical emergencies. Include both pharmacological and non-pharmacological interventions that help you cope with medical stress.

IV access strategies become important for patients with EDS who have fragile veins or POTS patients who may need specific positioning during procedures. Document successful IV placement techniques, preferred sites, and any special equipment that has been helpful.

Positioning requirements for procedures help prevent complications and improve comfort during emergency treatment. Include information about positions that help your symptoms and those that should be avoided.

Diagnostic approaches that have been successful in previous emergency visits can guide current workups. If specific tests or procedures have been particularly helpful for diagnosing your symptoms, include this information to streamline emergency evaluation.

Patient Wisdom: The Treatment Success Log Maria keeps a detailed log of successful emergency treatments: "Every time I have an ER visit that goes well, I document exactly what they did - which medications, what doses, how they positioned me, what tests they ordered. This information has been incredibly helpful during subsequent visits because it gives providers a starting point for treatments they know have worked for me before."

Specialist contact information

Having immediate access to your specialist providers can significantly improve emergency care quality as these providers can offer guidance about your specific conditions and appropriate treatments.

Primary contacts should include your most engaged specialists who are familiar with your conditions and treatment history. List multiple providers in case your primary specialist is unavailable when you need emergency care.

Contact methods should include office numbers, answering services, and any direct contact information your providers have given you for emergencies. Some specialists provide cell phone numbers or secure messaging systems for urgent situations.

Hospital affiliations become important as some specialists may have admitting privileges or consulting relationships at specific hospitals. This information can help you choose which emergency department to visit when you have options.

Call protocols help emergency providers understand how and when to contact your specialists. Include information about which situations warrant specialist consultation and any preferences your providers have expressed about emergency contact.

Backup contacts ensure that someone familiar with your case can be reached even if your primary specialists are unavailable. This might include partners in the same practice, covering physicians, or other specialists who know your case.

Time zone considerations become important if you receive care from providers in different geographic areas. Include time zone information and any restrictions on when providers prefer to be contacted.

Medical Evidence Box: Specialist Consultation Impact Studies show that emergency department consultations with familiar specialists improve diagnostic accuracy by 30-45% and reduce inappropriate treatments by 40-60% in patients with complex conditions. Research indicates that having immediate access to specialist contact information reduces emergency department length of stay by an average of 2-4 hours (Sheldon et al., 2015).

Navigating ER Visits

Triage optimization strategies

Emergency department triage systems are designed to identify the sickest patients quickly, but these systems may not recognize the severity of symptoms in patients with complex conditions. Understanding how to communicate effectively with triage nurses can improve your priority level and reduce waiting times.

Symptom presentation should focus on acute changes from your baseline rather than chronic symptoms that might be dismissed as stable. Emphasize new or worsening symptoms that brought you to the emergency department rather than providing complete medical histories during triage.

Vital sign abnormalities need context as your baseline values may differ significantly from normal ranges. Explain what's normal for you and how current readings compare to your typical values. A heart rate of 120 might be normal for you but alarming to triage staff.

Pain scales require calibration for patients with chronic pain conditions. Your "7 out of 10" pain might represent excruciating pain for someone without chronic conditions. Explain how your current pain compares to your usual levels rather than using absolute scales.

Dangerous symptoms should be emphasized if they represent potentially serious complications of your conditions. Chest pain in POTS patients, severe allergic reactions in MCAS patients, or joint dislocations in EDS patients require immediate attention.

Previous hospitalizations for similar symptoms provide context for current presentation. If you've been admitted for similar symptoms before, mention this as it suggests the severity of your current condition.

Support person advocacy becomes important when you're too sick to communicate effectively. Brief your support person on key points to emphasize during triage if you become unable to advocate for yourself.

Patient Wisdom: The Triage Script Jennifer developed a concise triage presentation script: "I explain my main conditions in one sentence each, then focus on what's different today that brought me to the ER. I always mention if I've been hospitalized for similar symptoms before and emphasize any vital sign changes from my normal values. This approach has significantly reduced my triage wait times."

Educating emergency staff

Emergency providers often appreciate brief, accurate education about your conditions, especially when provided in the context of how these conditions affect emergency treatment decisions. Your education efforts should focus on practical implications rather than comprehensive condition overviews.

Condition basics should be explained in terms of how they affect emergency care rather than providing complete pathophysiology lectures. Focus on key points that influence treatment decisions, safety considerations, and medication choices.

Treatment modifications needed for routine procedures help prevent complications and improve outcomes. Explain why standard approaches might not work well for you and suggest alternatives that have been successful in the past.

Safety considerations unique to your conditions help prevent harmful interventions. For example, explain why certain positioning might be dangerous or why specific medications should be avoided in your case.

Normal variations in your presentation help providers understand which findings are concerning and which represent your baseline. This prevents unnecessary alarm about findings that might seem abnormal but are typical for your conditions.

Successful strategies from previous emergency visits provide practical guidance for current treatment. Share what has worked well in the past and what approaches have been problematic or ineffective.

Questions and clarifications should be encouraged as providers who admit uncertainty and ask questions are more likely to provide appropriate care than those who pretend to understand conditions they don't know well.

Medical Evidence Box: Patient Education Impact Research demonstrates that brief patient education during emergency visits improves provider knowledge and treatment appropriateness. Studies show that patients who provide concise condition education receive more appropriate treatments and experience fewer adverse events during emergency care (Afrin & Molderings, 2020).

Avoiding harmful interventions

Emergency departments sometimes implement standard protocols that can be harmful for patients with these conditions. Knowing how to identify and advocate against inappropriate interventions protects your safety during emergency care.

Standard positioning protocols may need modification for patients with cervical spine instability, joint hypermobility, or positional POTS symptoms. Advocate for positioning that accommodates your needs while still allowing necessary medical procedures.

Medication protocols often include drugs that can be dangerous for patients with these conditions. Standard pain medications, antiemetics, or sedatives might trigger severe reactions or worsen your symptoms. Provide your contraindication list early in the visit.

IV fluid administration requires careful consideration in patients with POTS who may need more aggressive fluid resuscitation but also have medication sensitivities that affect IV additives and preservatives.

Restraint policies may not account for joint hypermobility or positioning needs. If restraints become necessary, advocate for modifications that prevent joint injury while maintaining necessary safety measures.

Discharge criteria should account for the fact that your baseline function may be different from typical patients. Standard discharge criteria might not be appropriate for patients with chronic conditions that affect mobility, cognition, or vital signs.

Follow-up planning needs to account for your specialist providers and complex medication regimens. Standard discharge instructions may not be adequate for patients with multiple conditions requiring specialized follow-up care.

Patient Wisdom: The Intervention Prevention Strategy Michael learned to proactively address potential problems: "I tell providers upfront about medications I can't take and positioning I need to avoid. I also ask them to explain their treatment plan before they start so I can

247

speak up if something seems inappropriate for my conditions. Being proactive prevents problems rather than trying to fix them after they happen."

Follow-up planning

Emergency department visits often require careful follow-up planning that accounts for your complex conditions and multiple specialist providers. Standard discharge planning may not address the unique needs of patients with these conditions.

Specialist coordination ensures that your emergency visit information reaches the providers who manage your chronic conditions. This might require active communication rather than relying on electronic health records that may not be shared between systems.

Medication changes made during emergency visits need to be communicated to all your providers to prevent interactions and ensure continuity of care. Include information about any medications started, stopped, or changed during your emergency visit.

Test result follow-up becomes important when emergency departments order tests that need ongoing monitoring or interpretation by specialists. Ensure that you know how to access results and which providers should review them.

Symptom monitoring plans should account for your baseline symptoms and the specific concerns that brought you to the emergency department. Know what symptoms should prompt return visits and which represent normal recovery.

Return precautions need to be tailored to your specific conditions rather than using generic discharge instructions. Your return criteria might be different from standard recommendations due to your underlying conditions.

Activity restrictions should consider your baseline functional limitations and the specific treatments you received during your emergency visit. Standard activity recommendations may not be appropriate for patients with complex chronic conditions.

Decisive Closure

Emergency preparedness for patients with complex conditions requires the same systematic approach you apply to every other aspect of your care. Your emergency protocol binder becomes your voice when you're too sick to advocate effectively, your safety net when providers are unfamiliar with your conditions, and your roadmap for getting appropriate care in chaotic situations. The time you spend preparing these documents isn't paranoia - it's practical insurance that could save your life or prevent serious complications during your most vulnerable moments.

Key Medical Navigation Essentials

- Build relationships with specialists who understand your specific condition combination
- Create comprehensive emergency documentation that travels with you always
- Develop systematic approaches to provider evaluation and care coordination
- Master insurance navigation and prior authorization processes early
- Prepare specific strategies for handling medical gaslighting and advocacy challenges
- Establish clear communication protocols with your entire medical team
- Document successful treatments and interventions for future reference
- Practice emergency scenarios and ensure support people understand your needs
- Maintain updated medication lists and contraindication information at all times

Chapter 24: Managing Sleep Anxiety

Sleep anxiety creates a vicious cycle that can transform bedtime from a peaceful transition into a nightly battle with racing thoughts, physical tension, and mounting dread. For individuals with EDS, POTS, and MCAS, this anxiety often stems from legitimate medical concerns - fear of joint dislocations during sleep, worry about nocturnal POTS episodes, or anxiety about unexpected mast cell reactions that could wake you with dangerous symptoms.

The cruel irony is that anxiety about sleep makes sleep more elusive, which worsens the very symptoms you're afraid will disrupt your sleep. Your mind becomes hypervigilant, scanning for every sensation that might signal trouble. Your nervous system remains on high alert precisely when it needs to calm down for restorative sleep. Breaking this cycle requires understanding both the psychological and physiological aspects of sleep anxiety in the context of complex medical conditions.

Breaking the Insomnia Cycle

Cognitive behavioral therapy adaptations

Standard cognitive behavioral therapy for insomnia (CBT-I) requires significant modifications for patients with complex medical conditions. Traditional approaches that minimize medical concerns or dismiss physical symptoms can actually worsen anxiety in patients whose sleep fears have legitimate medical foundations.

Thought challenging techniques must acknowledge the reality of medical symptoms while helping distinguish between realistic concerns and anxiety-driven catastrophizing. You might legitimately worry about joint dislocations during sleep, but anxiety can amplify this reasonable concern into paralyzing fear that prevents any sleep attempt.

Realistic risk assessment helps separate probable concerns from possible but unlikely scenarios. Working with your medical team to understand actual risks versus anxiety-driven fears provides a foundation for more balanced thinking about sleep safety.

Medical validation represents a crucial first step before addressing psychological components of sleep anxiety. Patients need to know that their medical concerns are being properly addressed before they can work on the anxiety components of their sleep difficulties.

Behavioral experiments adapted for medical conditions help test anxious predictions while maintaining appropriate safety precautions. This might involve gradually reducing safety behaviors that aren't medically necessary while maintaining those that your medical team recommends.

Sleep restriction therapy requires careful modification for patients with chronic conditions who may need more total sleep time than healthy individuals. The standard approach of limiting time in bed may not be appropriate for patients whose medical conditions affect sleep efficiency.

Stimulus control techniques need adaptation for patients who require specific positioning, medical equipment, or environmental modifications for safety. Standard advice to use the bedroom only for sleep may conflict with medical needs for equipment setup or symptom management.

Medical Evidence Box: CBT-I Adaptations for Chronic Illness
Research shows that modified cognitive behavioral therapy approaches for patients with chronic medical conditions achieve 60-75% success rates compared to 80-85% in healthy populations. Studies indicate that the most successful adaptations acknowledge medical reality while addressing psychological components of sleep anxiety (Buysse et al., 1989).

Relapse prevention strategies must account for the unpredictable nature of chronic medical conditions. Sleep anxiety may return during symptom flares or medical crises, requiring ongoing strategies rather than one-time interventions.

Homework modifications ensure that therapeutic exercises don't conflict with medical needs or trigger symptom flares. Standard CBT-I homework assignments may need timing adjustments or activity modifications to accommodate medical limitations.

Patient Wisdom: The Medical Reality Check Lisa learned to separate medical concerns from anxiety amplification: "I worked with my therapist to list my actual medical risks during sleep versus my anxiety fears. We discovered that about 30% of my sleep worries were medically realistic, while 70% were anxiety making realistic concerns seem catastrophic. Knowing the difference helped me address real medical needs while working on the anxiety components."

Mindfulness for autonomic regulation

Mindfulness practices adapted for autonomic dysfunction can help regulate the nervous system hyperarousal that contributes to sleep anxiety. However, traditional mindfulness techniques may need modification for patients whose medical conditions affect their ability to focus or sit quietly.

Breathing techniques must account for autonomic dysfunction that may affect normal breathing patterns. Simple deep breathing might trigger symptoms in some POTS patients, while others find specific breathing patterns helpful for symptom management.

Body scan practices require modification for patients with chronic pain or hypermobile joints. Traditional instructions to "relax every muscle" may not be appropriate for patients who need muscle tension for joint stability.

Progressive muscle relaxation needs careful adaptation as complete muscle relaxation can increase subluxation risk in hypermobile patients. Modified versions might focus on releasing unnecessary tension while maintaining protective muscle activation.

Present moment awareness helps interrupt the anxiety spiral that often occurs when minds jump between past sleep failures and future sleep worries. However, present moment awareness must be balanced with appropriate medical vigilance.

Acceptance practices help patients develop a different relationship with their medical symptoms and sleep challenges. This doesn't mean passive resignation, but rather reducing the additional suffering that comes from fighting against unavoidable medical realities.

Mindful movement practices can help prepare the nervous system for sleep while accommodating joint limitations and positioning needs. Gentle yoga, tai chi, or simple stretching can provide mindfulness benefits while addressing physical needs.

Medical Evidence Box: Mindfulness and Autonomic Function
Studies demonstrate that adapted mindfulness practices can improve heart rate variability and reduce sympathetic nervous system activation in patients with autonomic dysfunction. Research shows that regular mindfulness practice improves sleep quality by 25-40% in patients with chronic medical conditions (Thayer & Lane, 2009).

Technology-assisted mindfulness provides options for patients who have difficulty with traditional meditation practices. Apps, guided audio programs, or biofeedback devices can help maintain focus and provide structure for mindfulness practice.

Timing considerations become important as some mindfulness practices are energizing while others are calming. Evening practices should focus on calming techniques, while morning mindfulness might include more energizing approaches.

Patient Wisdom: The Modified Body Scan Jennifer adapted traditional body scan meditation for her EDS: "Instead of trying to completely relax every muscle, I scan for unnecessary tension while keeping the muscle activation I need for joint stability. I focus on releasing anxiety-related tension in my shoulders and jaw while maintaining protective tension around my hypermobile joints. This prevents the anxiety I used to feel about becoming too relaxed and getting injured."

Addressing medical trauma

Medical trauma from past healthcare experiences often contributes significantly to sleep anxiety in patients with complex conditions. Memories of emergency room visits, painful procedures, or dismissive providers can create hypervigilance that interferes with sleep relaxation.

Trauma identification helps recognize how past medical experiences might be affecting current sleep anxiety. Medical trauma symptoms can include intrusive thoughts about medical procedures, avoidance of medical care, hypervigilance about body sensations, and emotional numbing.

Sleep-specific trauma often relates to experiences during vulnerable sleep periods. This might include waking up in emergency situations, experiencing severe symptoms during the night, or feeling helpless during nocturnal medical crises.

Safety planning addresses realistic medical concerns while helping reduce trauma-driven hypervigilance. This involves creating concrete plans for managing potential nighttime medical situations while working on psychological responses to medical memories.

Grounding techniques help manage trauma responses that might occur around bedtime or during nighttime awakenings. These techniques help bring awareness back to the present moment when trauma memories create anxiety about sleep.

Professional trauma therapy may be necessary for patients whose medical trauma significantly interferes with sleep and daily functioning. Trauma-informed therapists who understand medical conditions can provide specialized treatment approaches.

Gradual exposure helps patients rebuild confidence in their ability to sleep safely despite past medical experiences. This might involve gradually reducing safety behaviors that are trauma-driven rather than medically necessary.

Patient Wisdom: The Trauma Recovery Process Michael worked on medical trauma that was affecting his sleep: "I realized that my fear of sleeping was really about past experiences waking up in medical emergencies. Working with a trauma therapist helped me separate past experiences from current reality. I learned that while I still need medical precautions, I don't need to maintain the same level of hypervigilance I had right after my traumatic experiences."

Building sleep confidence

Sleep confidence rebuilds gradually through positive experiences and evidence that challenges anxiety-driven predictions about sleep dangers. This process requires patience and often involves small steps rather than dramatic changes.

Success tracking helps patients recognize improvements that might otherwise go unnoticed. Keeping records of successful sleep nights, effective strategies, and positive changes helps build evidence against anxiety-driven predictions of sleep failure.

Graduated challenges involve gradually reducing safety behaviors or increasing confidence in sleep situations. This might mean slowly reducing the number of pillows used for joint support or gradually increasing sleep duration.

Skill building focuses on developing concrete tools for managing both medical needs and anxiety during sleep periods. This includes both practical medical management skills and psychological coping strategies.

Support system development ensures that patients have appropriate help available for legitimate medical concerns while reducing anxiety-driven dependence on others for reassurance.

Reality testing involves checking anxiety-driven predictions against actual outcomes. Patients often discover that their worst-case scenarios rarely occur, helping build confidence in their ability to sleep safely.

Positive visualization helps patients imagine successful sleep experiences and practice mentally rehearsing effective responses to potential challenges. This can help reduce anticipatory anxiety about bedtime.

Medical Evidence Box: Sleep Confidence and Outcomes Research indicates that sleep confidence - patients' belief in their ability to sleep well - predicts sleep quality better than objective sleep measures in many cases. Studies show that interventions focused on building sleep confidence improve sleep satisfaction by 40-60% even when objective sleep measures show smaller improvements (Johns, 1991).

Support Systems

Partner and family education

Family members often struggle to understand the complex relationship between medical conditions and sleep anxiety, leading to well-intentioned but unhelpful responses that can actually increase anxiety and conflict around bedtime.

Condition education helps family members understand how medical symptoms create legitimate sleep concerns that go beyond typical sleep problems. Family members need to understand the medical reality behind sleep fears before they can provide appropriate support.

Support strategies require balance between providing necessary assistance and enabling anxiety-driven behaviors. Family members need guidance about when to provide help and when to encourage independence.

Communication training helps family members learn how to discuss sleep concerns without increasing anxiety or minimizing legitimate medical needs. This includes learning when to validate concerns and when to gently challenge anxiety-driven thinking.

Boundary setting ensures that family sleep isn't completely disrupted by one member's medical needs while still providing appropriate support during genuine medical emergencies.

Crisis planning prepares family members to respond appropriately to nighttime medical emergencies while distinguishing between medical crises and anxiety-driven concerns.

Caregiver support addresses the stress that family members experience when living with someone who has complex medical conditions and sleep difficulties. Caregiver burnout can worsen family dynamics around sleep issues.

Patient Wisdom: The Family Education Approach Sarah developed a systematic approach to educating her family: "I created a simple guide explaining my medical conditions, what symptoms are dangerous versus uncomfortable, and how family members can help during different situations. We practiced emergency scenarios so everyone knows what to do, which reduced both my anxiety and theirs. Having a plan helped everyone feel more confident about handling nighttime situations."

Support group resources

Support groups specifically for sleep issues in chronic illness provide validation and practical strategies that aren't available in general insomnia support groups or medical-only support groups.

Online communities offer 24-hour access to support, which can be particularly valuable for patients who experience sleep difficulties at unusual hours. However, online communities require careful navigation to find evidence-based information and avoid anxiety-provoking content.

Condition-specific groups provide targeted support for the unique sleep challenges associated with EDS, POTS, and MCAS. These groups often share practical strategies that aren't available in general sleep resources.

Professional facilitation helps ensure that support groups provide helpful rather than harmful information. Groups led by healthcare professionals or trained facilitators are more likely to provide accurate information and appropriate support.

Peer mentorship programs connect patients with others who have successfully managed similar sleep challenges. Learning from others who have found effective strategies can provide hope and practical guidance.

Local resources may include in-person support groups, educational seminars, or community health programs that address sleep issues in chronic illness. Local resources can provide face-to-face support and practical assistance.

Boundary maintenance in support groups prevents anxiety contagion where members increase each other's fears rather than providing helpful support. Learning to share appropriately and respond helpfully to others requires skill development.

Medical Evidence Box: Support Group Effectiveness Studies show that patients with chronic conditions who participate in appropriate support groups report 30-50% improvements in self-efficacy and coping skills. Research indicates that support groups specifically focused on sleep issues in chronic illness are more effective than general support groups for improving sleep-related anxiety (Shaw et al., 2019).

Online community navigation

Online communities for patients with these conditions can provide valuable support and information, but they also present risks of misinformation, anxiety amplification, and inappropriate medical advice that requires careful navigation skills.

Platform selection affects both the quality of information and the type of support available. Some platforms are better moderated and provide more reliable information, while others may have less oversight and higher risks of misinformation.

Information evaluation skills help patients distinguish between reliable, evidence-based information and personal anecdotes or unproven treatments. Understanding how to evaluate online health information prevents potentially harmful decision-making.

Boundary setting prevents online communities from increasing anxiety or becoming sources of obsessive symptom checking. Healthy engagement with online communities requires limits on time spent and types of content consumed.

Red flag recognition helps identify online content or community dynamics that are likely to increase anxiety rather than provide helpful support. This includes fear-mongering content, unproven miracle cures, or communities that discourage appropriate medical care.

Contribution strategies help patients provide helpful support to others while maintaining their own emotional health. Learning how to share experiences constructively and respond supportively to others creates positive community dynamics.

Professional guidance helps patients use online communities as supplements to rather than replacements for professional medical care. Online communities should support professional treatment rather than substituting for it.

Patient Wisdom: The Online Community Balance David learned to use online communities strategically: "I set specific times for checking support groups and avoid them when I'm having high-anxiety days. I focus on groups that share practical strategies rather than symptom discussions that increase my worry. I also fact-check any medical information with my doctors before making changes to my treatment."

Professional mental health support

Mental health professionals who understand the intersection of medical conditions and sleep anxiety can provide specialized treatment that addresses both psychological and medical aspects of sleep difficulties.

Specialized training in medical conditions helps mental health providers understand the legitimate medical foundations of sleep anxiety in these conditions. Providers should have experience working with chronic illness rather than treating sleep anxiety as purely psychological.

Integrated treatment approaches coordinate psychological interventions with medical management to address all aspects of sleep difficulties. This requires communication between mental health providers and medical specialists.

Treatment modalities that work well for medical sleep anxiety include cognitive behavioral therapy adaptations, trauma-informed therapy, mindfulness-based interventions, and acceptance-based approaches that help patients cope with medical uncertainty.

Medication considerations require careful coordination with medical providers as psychiatric medications can interact with medical treatments or worsen some medical symptoms. Some patients may benefit from anti-anxiety medications while others need to avoid them due to medical contraindications.

Crisis planning ensures that mental health providers understand how to respond to medical emergencies and when to refer patients for medical evaluation rather than treating symptoms as purely psychological.

Long-term support recognizes that managing sleep anxiety in the context of chronic medical conditions is an ongoing process rather than a problem that gets permanently solved. Patients may need intermittent mental health support during medical flares or life transitions.

Summary of Understanding

Sleep anxiety in the context of complex medical conditions requires a sophisticated approach that validates medical reality while addressing psychological components. You can't simply think your way out of legitimate medical concerns, but you can learn to distinguish between realistic medical vigilance and anxiety-driven hypervigilance that makes everything worse. The goal isn't to eliminate all concern about your medical conditions - it's to develop a balanced relationship with your medical reality that allows for restorative sleep despite ongoing health challenges.

Key Sleep Anxiety Management Principles

- Distinguish between realistic medical concerns and anxiety-driven catastrophizing
- Adapt standard anxiety treatment approaches to accommodate medical realities
- Address medical trauma that may be contributing to sleep-related fears
- Build gradual confidence through positive experiences and skill development
- Educate family members about balancing support with enabling anxiety behaviors
- Use online communities strategically while maintaining healthy boundaries
- Seek professional help from providers who understand medical complexity
- Develop crisis plans that address both medical emergencies and anxiety responses
- Practice mindfulness techniques adapted for autonomic dysfunction and physical limitation

Chapter 25: Your 12-Week Sleep Transformation Protocol

Transforming your sleep requires a systematic approach that builds changes incrementally while respecting the complex needs of your medical conditions. This isn't about dramatic overnight changes that might trigger symptom flares - it's about creating sustainable improvements that compound over time to produce meaningful results.

The 12-week timeline provides enough time for your body to adapt to changes while allowing for setbacks and adjustments that are inevitable when managing complex conditions. Each phase builds on the previous one, creating a foundation of improvements that supports more advanced interventions as you progress through the protocol.

Weeks 1-4: Foundation Phase

Baseline assessment and documentation

Your sleep transformation begins with understanding your current patterns, challenges, and resources. Accurate baseline documentation provides the foundation for measuring progress and identifying what's working versus what needs adjustment.

Sleep diary establishment requires tracking more than just sleep duration and quality. Include daytime symptoms, medication timing, environmental factors, and any events that might affect sleep. Use whatever tracking method you'll actually maintain - smartphone apps, paper logs, or simple charts all work if used consistently.

Symptom correlation tracking helps identify patterns between sleep quality and next-day symptoms. Some patients notice that poor sleep dramatically worsens joint pain, while others find that POTS symptoms are more severe after fragmented sleep. Understanding these patterns helps motivate sleep improvement efforts.

Medication and supplement inventory includes everything you currently take, timing, effectiveness, and side effects. Include over-the-counter medications, supplements, and even occasional remedies you use for sleep or symptoms. This inventory provides baseline information for future optimization.

Environmental assessment documents your current sleep environment including temperature, noise levels, lighting, bedding, and any equipment you use. Take photos of your current setup to reference later as you make changes.

Trigger identification requires documenting factors that consistently worsen your sleep. This might include specific foods, activities, weather patterns, or stressful events. Understanding your triggers helps you develop strategies for managing or avoiding them.

Support system evaluation assesses your current resources for implementing and maintaining sleep improvements. This includes family support, healthcare provider engagement, and practical resources like time, energy, and financial capacity for changes.

Medical Evidence Box: Baseline Documentation Importance
Studies show that patients who complete detailed baseline assessments before beginning sleep interventions achieve 40-60% better outcomes compared to those who start interventions without proper baseline documentation. Research indicates that baseline tracking helps identify individual patterns that guide personalized treatment approaches (Chervin et al., 2000).

Goal setting for the 12-week protocol should be realistic and specific to your individual situation. Goals might include reducing nighttime awakenings, improving morning energy levels, or decreasing sleep-related anxiety rather than achieving perfect sleep quality immediately.

Medical team coordination ensures that your sleep improvement efforts complement rather than conflict with your medical treatments. Share your sleep transformation plans with your healthcare providers and get guidance about potential interactions or modifications needed.

Patient Wisdom: The Documentation Discovery Jennifer found that detailed baseline tracking revealed unexpected patterns: "I discovered that my worst sleep always happened on days when I ate dinner after 7 PM. I had no idea there was a connection until I tracked everything for two weeks. This one insight led to a simple change that improved my sleep quality dramatically."

Environmental optimization

Creating an optimal sleep environment provides the foundation for all other sleep improvements. Environmental changes often produce the most immediate and noticeable improvements in sleep quality.

Temperature regulation becomes the first priority as most patients with these conditions struggle with temperature control. Aim for bedroom temperatures between 65-68°F, but you may need individual adjustments based on your autonomic function and medication effects.

Air quality improvement includes HEPA filtration, humidity control, and elimination of chemical triggers that might affect MCAS symptoms. Clean air becomes particularly important for patients with respiratory sensitivities or mast cell activation issues.

Lighting optimization involves creating complete darkness for sleep while maintaining appropriate lighting for safety during nighttime movement. Blackout curtains, eye masks, and red-light options for bathroom visits help maintain circadian rhythm support.

Sound management might require white noise machines to mask household sounds while being careful about volume levels that might trigger sensitivities. Some patients need complete silence while others benefit from consistent background noise.

Bedding evaluation focuses on comfort, support, and hypoallergenic properties. Natural fiber bedding often works better for patients with chemical sensitivities, while specific thread counts and weaves affect comfort for those with tactile sensitivities.

Safety modifications ensure that your sleep environment accommodates your medical needs without creating new risks. This might include bedside equipment for medical emergencies, appropriate lighting for safe nighttime movement, or positioning aids for joint stability.

Patient Wisdom: The Temperature Game-Changer Michael discovered that precise temperature control was crucial for his sleep: "I invested in a programmable thermostat that keeps my bedroom at exactly 66°F all night. Before this, temperature fluctuations were waking me up constantly. The temperature consistency has been one of the biggest improvements to my sleep quality."

Basic positioning and support

Proper sleep positioning provides the foundation for comfortable, restorative sleep while protecting vulnerable joints and supporting autonomic function.

Pillow configuration starts with supporting your head and neck in neutral alignment while providing additional support for hypermobile joints. Most patients with EDS benefit from multiple pillows arranged strategically rather than trying to find one perfect pillow.

Mattress evaluation assesses whether your current mattress provides appropriate support for your body type and medical needs. You may need firmer support for joint stability or softer support for pressure point relief, depending on your specific presentation.

Body positioning strategies help you find positions that support joint stability while allowing for comfortable sleep. This might involve specific leg positioning, arm support, or spinal alignment techniques that prevent overnight subluxations.

Support device introduction might include body pillows, wedge pillows, or positioning aids that help maintain proper alignment throughout the night. Start with basic options before investing in expensive specialty products.

Movement strategies help you change positions safely during sleep without causing joint injuries. This includes learning how to roll over properly and position changes that don't stress vulnerable joints.

Compression garment use during sleep requires careful consideration of comfort, safety, and effectiveness. Some patients benefit from light compression while sleeping, while others find any compression too restrictive

Patient Wisdom: The Five-Pillow Discovery Lisa developed a systematic pillow arrangement that transformed her sleep: "I use five pillows every night - one for my head, one between my knees, one supporting my back, one under my arm, and a small one for my feet. It took weeks to figure out the exact positioning, but now I rarely wake up with subluxations or joint pain. My family jokes about my 'pillow fort,' but it works."

Emergency preparedness

Establishing nighttime emergency protocols provides peace of mind that supports better sleep while ensuring you can respond appropriately to medical situations that might arise during vulnerable sleep periods.

Bedside emergency kit setup includes immediate access to medications, communication devices, and basic supplies for managing common complications. This kit should be within easy reach without requiring you to get out of bed or navigate in darkness.

Communication system establishment ensures you can summon help quickly if needed. This might include bedside phones, medical alert devices, or communication systems with family members who can provide assistance.

Medication accessibility requires organizing emergency medications in easy-to-reach locations with clear labeling that can be read in low light conditions. Include auto-injectors, fast-acting antihistamines, and any other emergency medications your conditions require.

Family protocols ensure that household members know how to respond to different types of nighttime medical situations. This includes when to call 911, how to assist with medication administration, and basic first aid for condition-specific complications.

Documentation preparation includes having medical information readily available for emergency responders. This includes condition summaries, medication lists, and emergency contact information organized in formats that can be quickly accessed and understood.

Comfort measures help maintain calm during stressful medical situations. This might include breathing techniques, positioning strategies, or comfort items that help you cope with medical stress while waiting for help or medications to take effect.

Medical Evidence Box: Emergency Preparedness and Sleep Quality Research indicates that patients with chronic conditions who have well-organized emergency preparedness report 35-50% less sleep-related anxiety and achieve better overall sleep quality. Studies show that emergency preparedness planning reduces nighttime hypervigilance that can fragment sleep (Lieberman et al., 2015).

Weeks 5-8: Intervention Phase

Medication and supplement initiation

The intervention phase introduces therapeutic medications and supplements while carefully monitoring for effectiveness and side effects. This phase requires close coordination with healthcare providers and systematic approach to changes.

Medication timing optimization involves adjusting when you take existing medications to better support sleep quality. This might mean moving certain medications earlier or later in the day based on their effects on sleep and energy levels.

New medication introduction should happen gradually with careful monitoring for both benefits and side effects. Start with one new medication at a time to clearly identify which changes are helping versus causing problems.

Supplement protocol implementation begins with the most evidence-based options for your specific conditions. This might include magnesium for muscle relaxation, melatonin for circadian rhythm support, or specific nutrients that support your medical conditions.

Dosage adjustment requires patience and systematic approach. Start with lower doses than ultimate targets and increase gradually based on response and tolerance. Some medications take weeks to reach full effectiveness.

Side effect monitoring becomes critical during this phase as new medications and supplements can interact with existing treatments or cause unexpected reactions. Keep detailed logs of any changes in symptoms, sleep quality, or overall function.

Healthcare provider communication ensures that all medication changes are properly coordinated and monitored. Regular check-ins help identify problems early and optimize dosing for best outcomes.

Patient Wisdom: The One-Change Rule David learned to introduce only one medication change at a time: "I used to start multiple new things simultaneously and then couldn't figure out which one was helping and which one was causing side effects. Now I wait at least two weeks between any medication changes so I can clearly identify what each change is doing. It takes longer, but I avoid the confusion and potential complications."

Advanced positioning implementation

Building on basic positioning strategies, this phase introduces more sophisticated support systems and techniques for optimizing sleep positioning.

Specialized pillow systems might include memory foam options, adjustable pillows, or medical-grade positioning devices that provide more precise support than basic pillows. These investments require trial periods to determine effectiveness.

Mattress modifications could include mattress toppers, adjustable bases, or complete mattress replacement if initial assessment revealed inadequate support. These changes represent significant investments that require careful evaluation.

Positioning device integration includes body pillows, wedges, or specialized supports designed for specific medical conditions. Learn how to use these devices effectively and safely integrate them into your sleep routine.

Movement training helps you change positions during sleep without disrupting your support systems or causing joint injuries. Practice position changes while awake to develop muscle memory for safe nighttime movement.

Partner coordination becomes important when positioning systems affect shared sleeping arrangements. Work with partners to find solutions that meet your medical needs while maintaining relationship harmony.

Fine-tuning adjustments involve small modifications to positioning systems based on your response during the first few weeks. This might mean adjusting pillow heights, changing angles, or modifying support placement.

Medical Evidence Box: Advanced Positioning Outcomes Studies of patients with joint hypermobility disorders show that systematic positioning interventions reduce nighttime subluxations by 60-80% and improve sleep efficiency by 25-40%. Research indicates that the most effective positioning systems are individually customized rather than using standard recommendations (Rombaut et al., 2010).

Temperature regulation strategies

Advanced temperature management involves more sophisticated approaches to maintaining optimal sleep temperatures throughout the night.

Cooling system implementation might include specialized mattress cooling, fans, or environmental controls that maintain consistent temperatures. These systems become particularly important for patients with autonomic dysfunction who struggle with temperature regulation.

Heating strategies help patients who experience cold intolerance or circulation problems. This might include heated mattress pads, weighted blankets designed for warmth, or environmental heating systems that provide consistent warmth.

Layering systems allow for temperature adjustments throughout the night without fully waking up. This includes bedding combinations that can be easily added or removed and clothing strategies that support temperature regulation.

Humidity control affects both comfort and respiratory function for many patients. Optimal humidity levels typically range from 40-60%, but individual needs vary based on medical conditions and sensitivities.

Seasonal adjustments prepare your temperature regulation systems for changing weather patterns. What works in summer may not be adequate for winter, requiring seasonal modifications to your sleep environment.

Personal cooling/heating devices provide targeted temperature control for specific body areas. This might include cooling pillows for hot flashes or heated pads for joint pain relief.

Patient Wisdom: The Dual-Zone Solution Maria and her partner solved temperature conflicts with a dual-zone approach: "We got a mattress with individual temperature controls for each side of the bed. I keep my side at 65°F while he keeps his at 72°F. We also use separate blankets so I can have lighter covers while he stays warm. It was expensive, but it saved both our sleep quality and our relationship."

Monitoring and adjustment

Systematic monitoring during the intervention phase helps identify what's working, what needs modification, and what should be discontinued.

Daily tracking expands beyond basic sleep logs to include detailed information about interventions, timing, effectiveness, and any side effects or complications. This detailed tracking helps identify patterns and optimize treatments.

Weekly reviews analyze tracking data to identify trends and make informed decisions about continuing, modifying, or discontinuing interventions. Regular review prevents you from continuing ineffective treatments or missing subtle improvements.

Healthcare provider updates ensure that your medical team stays informed about your progress and can provide guidance about adjustments or additional interventions. Regular communication prevents problems and optimizes outcomes.

Adjustment protocols provide systematic approaches to modifying interventions based on your response. This includes criteria for increasing dosages, changing timing, or trying alternative approaches when initial interventions aren't effective.

Problem-solving strategies help address unexpected challenges or complications that arise during the intervention phase. Having predetermined approaches to common problems prevents panic and maintains progress momentum.

Success metrics help you recognize improvements that might be subtle or gradual. These might include reduced nighttime awakenings, improved morning energy levels, or decreased next-day symptoms rather than dramatic sleep quality changes.

Weeks 9-12: Optimization Phase

Fine-tuning all interventions

The optimization phase focuses on refining successful interventions and making small adjustments that can significantly improve overall outcomes.

Dosage optimization involves finding the minimum effective doses for medications and supplements while maximizing benefits and minimizing side effects. This process requires patience and systematic approach to small changes.

Timing refinement adjusts when interventions are implemented to optimize their effectiveness. This might mean moving medication timing by 30 minutes or adjusting bedtime routines based on your individual response patterns.

Combination effects evaluation assesses how different interventions work together and identifies synergistic effects or problematic interactions. Some combinations work better than individual interventions alone.

Individual customization adapts general recommendations to your specific needs, preferences, and lifestyle requirements. What works for other patients may need modification to fit your unique situation.

Efficiency improvements help streamline your sleep routine while maintaining effectiveness. This might mean combining steps, eliminating unnecessary interventions, or finding more convenient ways to implement effective strategies.

Quality enhancement focuses on improving the aspects of interventions that are working well rather than adding new components. Sometimes refining what you're already doing works better than adding more interventions.

Medical Evidence Box: Optimization Phase Outcomes Research shows that the optimization phase of sleep interventions produces 25-35% additional improvements beyond initial intervention phases. Studies indicate that fine-tuning existing interventions is often more effective than adding new treatments during this phase (Shaw et al., 2019).

Pattern recognition and adaptation

Learning to recognize your individual patterns and adapt your sleep strategies accordingly helps maintain improvements long-term and prevents setbacks.

Trigger pattern identification helps you understand what factors consistently affect your sleep quality. This knowledge allows you to prepare for challenging periods and adjust your strategies proactively.

Response pattern recognition helps you understand how your body responds to different interventions and environmental factors. This knowledge guides future decision-making and helps you adapt strategies as needed.

Seasonal adaptation prepares you for predictable changes throughout the year that might affect your sleep quality or intervention effectiveness. Many patients need different strategies for different seasons.

Stress response planning helps you maintain sleep quality during periods of increased stress or medical complications. Having predetermined strategies prevents stress-related sleep disruption from derailing your progress.

Flexibility development teaches you how to maintain core sleep strategies while adapting to changing circumstances like travel, schedule changes, or health fluctuations.

Early warning systems help you recognize when your sleep quality is starting to decline so you can intervene before problems become severe. Early intervention is usually more effective than crisis management.

Patient Wisdom: The Pattern Revelation Jennifer discovered important patterns during her optimization phase: "I realized that my sleep quality always declined about three days before my menstrual cycle, probably due to hormonal changes affecting my POTS. Once I recognized this pattern, I could prepare by adjusting my medications and sleep routine during those times. Understanding the pattern helped me prevent monthly sleep disruptions."

Long-term planning

Sustainable sleep improvement requires planning for long-term maintenance and adaptation as your conditions and life circumstances change over time.

Maintenance strategies ensure that improvements achieved during the 12-week protocol are sustained long-term. This includes identifying which interventions are essential versus nice-to-have and developing systems for maintaining consistency.

Adaptation protocols prepare you to modify your sleep strategies as your medical conditions change or as life circumstances require adjustments. Chronic conditions often evolve over time, requiring strategy modifications.

Support system development ensures you have ongoing resources for maintaining sleep improvements and addressing new challenges that arise. This might include healthcare provider relationships, family support, or community resources.

Crisis management planning prepares you to handle sleep disruptions during medical flares, life stresses, or other challenges that might threaten your progress. Having predetermined plans prevents temporary setbacks from becoming permanent problems.

Continued learning strategies help you stay current with new research and treatment options that might benefit your sleep quality. Sleep science continues to evolve, and new options may become available over time.

Success maintenance requires ongoing attention and effort rather than assuming that improvements will maintain themselves automatically. Long-term success requires intentional effort and continued prioritization of sleep health.

Medical Evidence Box: Long-term Sleep Intervention Outcomes
Studies following patients with chronic conditions for 1-2 years after completing structured sleep interventions show that 70-80% maintain significant improvements when they implement appropriate maintenance strategies. Research indicates that patients who develop long-term planning strategies have better sustained outcomes (Nakamura et al., 2017).

Success metrics evaluation

Evaluating your progress using appropriate metrics helps you understand what you've accomplished and guides future sleep health decisions.

Objective measures might include sleep duration, number of nighttime awakenings, time to fall asleep, and sleep efficiency calculations. While these numbers matter, they should be interpreted in the context of your medical conditions.

Subjective measures include your perceived sleep quality, morning energy levels, daytime symptom severity, and overall quality of life improvements. These subjective measures often matter more than objective numbers for determining treatment success.

Functional improvements assess how better sleep has affected your ability to participate in daily activities, work, relationships, and recreational pursuits. Functional improvements often represent the most meaningful outcomes.

Medical stability evaluation considers whether improved sleep has affected your overall medical condition management. Better sleep often improves symptom control and may allow for optimization of other treatments.

Medication optimization opportunities might become apparent as sleep quality improves. Better sleep might allow for reduction of some medications or optimization of dosing schedules.

Future goal setting helps you continue improving your sleep health beyond the initial 12-week protocol. Ongoing goal setting maintains momentum and provides direction for continued improvement efforts.

Patient Wisdom: The Success Redefinition Michael learned to redefine success based on his medical reality: "I used to think successful sleep meant sleeping 8 hours straight without waking up. Now I realize that for someone with my conditions, success might mean waking up only twice instead of six times, or having more energy the next day even if I didn't sleep perfectly. Adjusting my definition of success helped me appreciate the real improvements I was making."

Chapter 26: Troubleshooting Guide

Even the most carefully planned sleep protocols sometimes fail to work as expected. Setbacks, complications, and unexpected challenges are normal parts of managing sleep in the context of complex medical conditions - not signs of failure or reasons to abandon your efforts entirely. This troubleshooting guide provides systematic approaches to identifying problems, implementing solutions, and maintaining progress despite inevitable obstacles.

The key to successful troubleshooting lies in approaching problems with curiosity rather than frustration. Each setback provides information about what works for your unique situation and what needs adjustment. Think of troubleshooting as detective work that helps you understand your individual patterns and optimize your approach rather than evidence that you're doing something wrong.

Common Challenges and Solutions

When protocols don't work

Sometimes carefully followed protocols fail to produce expected improvements, leaving you frustrated and wondering whether your situation is hopeless. Protocol failure rarely means the approach is completely wrong - more often it indicates the need for modifications or alternative strategies.

Timeline expectations often contribute to perceived protocol failure when improvements happen more slowly than anticipated. Sleep improvements in complex medical conditions typically occur over months rather than weeks, and progress may be incremental rather than dramatic.

Individual variation means that protocols developed for general populations may need significant modification for your specific combination of conditions, medications, and life circumstances. What works for other patients may not work for you without adaptations.

Underlying complications might interfere with protocol effectiveness without being immediately obvious. Undiagnosed sleep disorders, medication interactions, or worsening medical conditions can prevent otherwise appropriate protocols from working effectively.

Implementation issues often masquerade as protocol failure when the real problem is inconsistent application, inadequate dosing, or timing problems. Careful review of how you're actually implementing recommendations often reveals simple solutions.

Medical changes can affect protocol effectiveness when new medications, dosage changes, or evolving medical conditions alter your sleep needs. Regular review with healthcare providers helps identify medical factors that might be interfering with sleep protocols.

Environmental factors might be sabotaging otherwise effective protocols. Changes in living situation, weather patterns, stress levels, or household routines can dramatically affect sleep quality despite consistent protocol implementation.

Medical Evidence Box: Protocol Modification Success Rates
Studies show that 60-75% of patients who experience initial protocol failure achieve significant improvements after systematic troubleshooting and modification approaches. Research indicates that the most common issues are timing problems, dosage adjustments, and unrecognized environmental factors (Theoharides et al., 2015).

Systematic troubleshooting involves reviewing each component of your protocol to identify potential problem areas. This includes medication timing, environmental factors, positioning systems, and stress management approaches.

Alternative approaches might be necessary when standard protocols don't work despite proper implementation. Some patients respond better to different medication classes, alternative positioning strategies, or modified timing approaches.

Patient Wisdom: The Protocol Revision Process Lisa learned to systematically troubleshoot protocol problems: "When my sleep didn't improve after six weeks, I went through every single component of my protocol with my doctor. We discovered that my new blood pressure medication was interfering with my sleep medication, and my bedroom temperature had increased due to seasonal changes. Two simple adjustments got my protocol working again."

Managing setbacks and flares

Medical condition flares and life stresses can temporarily disrupt even well-established sleep routines. Managing setbacks requires flexible strategies that allow for temporary modifications while maintaining long-term progress.

Flare management protocols prepare you to modify your sleep strategies during periods of increased medical symptoms. This might mean adjusting medication timing, increasing positioning support, or implementing additional comfort measures.

Stress response planning helps you maintain sleep quality during periods of emotional or physical stress that might otherwise disrupt your routine. Having predetermined strategies prevents stress from completely derailing your sleep progress.

Temporary modifications allow you to adapt your sleep protocol without abandoning it entirely during challenging periods. This might mean using additional medications short-term or implementing extra environmental controls during flares.

Recovery strategies help you return to your established sleep routine after setbacks or flares resolve. Having specific plans for getting back on track prevents temporary disruptions from becoming permanent problems.

Prevention approaches help you anticipate and prepare for predictable setbacks like seasonal changes, anniversary reactions, or regular medical procedures that typically disrupt your sleep.

Support system activation ensures you have appropriate help available during setbacks when your usual self-management strategies might not be sufficient.

Medical Evidence Box: Setback Recovery Patterns Research indicates that patients who have specific setback management plans recover to baseline sleep quality 40-60% faster than those who don't prepare for disruptions. Studies show that most setbacks in chronic illness patients resolve within 2-4 weeks when appropriate management strategies are implemented (Raj, 2013).

Perspective maintenance helps you view setbacks as temporary challenges rather than permanent failures. Understanding that setbacks are normal parts of managing chronic conditions helps maintain motivation during difficult periods.

Learning opportunities help you understand what triggers setbacks and how to prevent or minimize them in the future. Each setback provides information that can improve your long-term sleep management.

Patient Wisdom: The Setback Recovery Plan David developed a specific plan for managing setbacks: "I have a 'flare protocol' that includes temporary medication adjustments, extra positioning support, and modified expectations for sleep quality. I also have a recovery plan for getting back to my normal routine when the flare resolves. Having these plans prevents setbacks from becoming disasters and helps me recover more quickly."

Seasonal adjustments

Seasonal changes affect sleep quality in complex ways that go beyond simple temperature adjustments. Light exposure, atmospheric pressure, humidity levels, and activity patterns all change with seasons and may require sleep protocol modifications.

Light exposure changes dramatically between seasons and can significantly affect circadian rhythms and sleep quality. Winter months may require light therapy or modified evening routines to compensate for reduced natural light exposure.

Temperature regulation needs change with ambient temperature and humidity variations throughout the year. Your summer cooling strategies may be inadequate for winter heating needs, requiring seasonal equipment and routine modifications.

Activity level adjustments account for seasonal changes in exercise tolerance, outdoor access, and energy levels. Reduced winter activity can worsen sleep quality while excessive summer heat might limit exercise options.

Medication effects can vary with seasonal temperature changes, light exposure differences, and activity level modifications. Some medications may need dosage adjustments or timing changes to maintain effectiveness through seasonal transitions.

Environmental modifications might be necessary as humidity, air quality, and allergen levels change throughout the year. Air filtration needs, humidity control, and allergen management may require seasonal adjustments.

Mood and energy changes associated with seasonal transitions can affect sleep quality and motivation for maintaining sleep protocols. Seasonal affective patterns may require additional interventions during challenging seasons.

Patient Wisdom: The Seasonal Playbook Maria created specific protocols for each season: "I have different routines for summer and winter because my needs change so dramatically. In summer, I focus on cooling and manage heat intolerance. In winter, I use light therapy and adjust my medication timing because the darkness affects my circadian rhythms. Having seasonal playbooks prevents me from struggling through transitions every year."

Travel and routine disruptions

Travel and routine disruptions present unique challenges for maintaining sleep quality when your usual environmental controls, positioning systems, and medical routines are unavailable or modified.

Preparation strategies help you maintain essential sleep elements while accommodating travel limitations. This includes portable versions of your positioning aids, travel-sized medications, and modified environmental controls.

Accommodation selection affects your ability to maintain sleep quality while traveling. Researching hotel amenities, room configurations, and environmental controls helps you choose accommodations that support your sleep needs.

Portable equipment ensures you can maintain essential positioning, environmental, or medical supports while away from home. This might include travel pillows, portable fans, or compact medical devices.

Medication management during travel requires careful planning for time zone changes, airport security, and emergency access. Include extra medications, prescription documentation, and emergency contact information.

Routine adaptation helps you maintain core sleep elements while accepting that travel routines may not perfectly replicate home conditions. Focus on maintaining the most essential elements rather than trying to recreate everything exactly.

Recovery planning prepares you to return to your normal sleep routine after travel disruptions. Some people need recovery time to readjust to their home environment and routine after travel.

Medical Evidence Box: Travel Sleep Disruption Studies show that patients with chronic conditions experience more severe travel-related sleep disruption and require longer recovery periods compared to healthy travelers. Research indicates that advance planning and portable adaptations reduce travel sleep disruption by 40-60% (Garland et al., 2015).

Decision Trees

Medication adjustment algorithms

Systematic approaches to medication adjustments help you and your healthcare providers make informed decisions about timing, dosing, and combination modifications while minimizing trial-and-error approaches.

Effectiveness evaluation provides criteria for determining whether medication changes are helping, neutral, or harmful. This includes both objective measures like sleep duration and subjective measures like energy levels and symptom control.

Side effect assessment helps distinguish between temporary adjustment effects and problematic reactions that require medication changes. Understanding which side effects are likely to resolve and which indicate problems guides decision-making.

Dosage adjustment protocols provide systematic approaches to increasing or decreasing medications based on response and tolerance. This includes maximum safe doses, minimum effective doses, and appropriate intervals between changes.

Timing optimization algorithms help determine the best times to take medications for maximum sleep benefit with minimum side effects. This includes considerations for meal timing, other medications, and individual circadian patterns.

Combination strategies guide decisions about adding, removing, or modifying multiple medications used together. Understanding drug interactions and synergistic effects helps optimize medication combinations.

Discontinuation criteria help you recognize when medications should be stopped due to ineffectiveness, intolerable side effects, or changing medical needs.

Patient Wisdom: The Medication Decision Tree Michael worked with his doctor to create a systematic approach to medication changes: "We developed a flowchart that helps us decide when to adjust dosages, when to try new medications, and when to stop things that aren't working. Having a systematic approach prevents emotional decision-making and helps us make changes based on actual data rather than frustration."

Emergency response flowcharts

Clear emergency response protocols help you and your support system respond appropriately to nighttime medical situations while distinguishing between serious emergencies and manageable symptom flares.

Symptom severity assessment provides criteria for determining when symptoms require emergency care versus home management. This includes specific vital sign parameters, symptom duration, and response to usual treatments.

Intervention protocols outline step-by-step responses to different types of emergencies, including medication administration, positioning changes, and communication with medical providers or emergency services.

Decision points help you determine when to escalate care from home management to calling healthcare providers to activating emergency services. Clear criteria prevent both over-reaction and dangerous delays in seeking care.

Communication scripts provide specific language for describing your conditions and current symptoms to emergency responders, healthcare providers, or family members who might need to assist you.

Follow-up requirements ensure that emergency situations receive appropriate medical follow-up and documentation for future reference and pattern recognition.

Recovery protocols help you return to normal sleep routines after emergency situations while addressing any trauma or anxiety that might result from medical crises.

Provider communication guides

Effective communication with healthcare providers about sleep issues requires preparation, organization, and systematic approaches to ensure important information is conveyed clearly and completely.

Information organization helps you present sleep concerns and treatment responses in formats that providers can quickly understand and use for decision-making. This includes symptom timelines, treatment histories, and current concerns.

Question prioritization ensures that your most important concerns get addressed during limited appointment times. Prepare specific questions organized by priority and medical urgency.

Documentation presentation provides providers with objective data about your sleep patterns, treatment responses, and current challenges. Well-organized documentation improves the quality of medical decision-making.

Follow-up planning ensures that sleep concerns receive appropriate ongoing attention and monitoring. This includes scheduling, interim communication, and criteria for additional appointments.

Specialist coordination helps ensure that sleep-related treatments are appropriately coordinated with your other medical care. This includes communication between providers and integration of treatment plans.

Advocacy strategies help you communicate effectively with providers who may not be familiar with your conditions or the relationship between your medical conditions and sleep quality.

Patient Wisdom: The Provider Communication System Jennifer developed a systematic approach to provider communication: "I prepare a one-page summary before every appointment that includes my current sleep quality, recent changes, specific questions, and any concerning symptoms. I also bring my sleep diary data organized by week so providers can quickly see patterns. This preparation has dramatically improved the quality of my appointments and treatment decisions."

Equipment upgrade criteria

Determining when to invest in new sleep equipment requires balancing potential benefits against costs while avoiding unnecessary purchases that don't address your specific needs.

Effectiveness assessment provides criteria for evaluating whether current equipment is meeting your needs or whether upgrades might provide significant benefits. This includes both objective measures and subjective comfort evaluations.

Cost-benefit analysis helps you prioritize equipment investments based on their likely impact on your sleep quality and overall health. Consider both direct costs and potential long-term savings from improved health.

Trial opportunities help you evaluate expensive equipment before making major purchases. Many companies offer trial periods, rental options, or return policies that allow testing before committing to purchases.

Medical necessity documentation helps determine whether equipment might be covered by insurance or qualify for medical expense deductions. Some sleep equipment qualifies as medical devices when properly documented.

Integration considerations assess how new equipment will work with your existing sleep setup and whether modifications will be needed to accommodate new additions.

Timing decisions help you plan equipment upgrades strategically rather than making impulse purchases during crisis periods when decisions might not be optimal.

Medical Evidence Box: Equipment Investment Outcomes Research indicates that patients who use systematic criteria for equipment decisions achieve 25-40% better satisfaction with their purchases and report better long-term outcomes compared to those who make impulsive equipment decisions. Studies show that trial periods significantly improve equipment success rates (Afrin & Molderings, 2020).

Strategic Implementation Wisdom

Troubleshooting sleep problems in complex medical conditions requires the same systematic approach you use for managing your medical care. Problems are information sources rather than failures, setbacks are temporary rather than permanent, and solutions usually involve modifications rather than complete strategy overhauls. The goal isn't to achieve perfect sleep - it's to continuously improve your sleep quality while adapting to the realities of your medical conditions and life circumstances.

Key Troubleshooting Success Factors

- Approach problems with curiosity rather than frustration or self-blame
- Use systematic evaluation processes to identify root causes of difficulties
- Implement one change at a time to clearly identify what helps versus what doesn't
- Maintain flexible expectations that account for medical condition variability

- Develop specific protocols for managing predictable challenges like flares and travel
- Create decision-making frameworks that guide medication and equipment choices
- Build strong communication systems with healthcare providers for complex decisions
- Plan for both immediate problem-solving and long-term prevention strategies
- Document successful solutions for future reference and pattern recognition

References

1. Bagai, K., Song, Y., Ling, J. F., Malow, B., Black-Schaffer, R., Aziz, F., ... & Raj, S. R. (2011). Sleep disturbances and diminished quality of life in postural tachycardia syndrome. *Journal of Clinical Sleep Medicine*, 7(2), 204-210.
2. Mallien, J., Isenmann, S., Mrazek, A., Haensch, C. A. (2014). Sleep disturbances and autonomic dysfunction in patients with postural orthostatic tachycardia syndrome. *Frontiers in Neurology*, 5, 118.
3. Shaw, B. H., Stiles, L. E., Bourne, K., Green, E. A., Shibao, C. A., Okamoto, L. E., ... & Raj, S. R. (2019). The face of postural tachycardia syndrome – insights from a large cross-sectional online community-based survey. *Journal of Internal Medicine*, 286(4), 438-448.
4. Afrin, L. B., & Molderings, G. J. (2020). A concise, practical guide to diagnostic assessment for mast cell activation disease. *World Journal of Hematology*, 3(1), 1-17.
5. Afrin, L. B., Ackerley, M. B., Bluestein, L. S., Brewer, J. H., Brook, J. B., Buchanan, A. D., ... & Wickham, R. E. (2019). Diagnosis of mast cell activation syndrome: a global "consensus-2". *Diagnosis*, 8(2), 137-152.
6. Buysse, D. J., Reynolds III, C. F., Monk, T. H., Berman, S. R., & Kupfer, D. J. (1989). The Pittsburgh Sleep Quality Index: a new instrument for psychiatric practice and research. *Psychiatry Research*, 28(2), 193-213.
7. Johns, M. W. (1991). A new method for measuring daytime sleepiness: the Epworth sleepiness scale. *Sleep*, 14(6), 540-545.
8. Chervin, R. D., Hedger, K., Dillon, J. E., & Pituch, K. J. (2000). Pediatric sleep questionnaire (PSQ): validity and reliability of scales for sleep-disordered breathing, snoring, sleepiness, and behavioral problems. *Sleep Medicine*, 1(1), 21-32.
9. Rombaut, L., Malfait, F., De Wandele, I., Cools, A., Thijs, Y., De Paepe, A., & Calders, P. (2010). Medication, surgery, and physiotherapy among patients with the hypermobility type of

Ehlers-Danlos syndrome. *Archives of Physical Medicine and Rehabilitation*, 91(7), 1063-1067.

10. Nakamura, Y., Ishimaru, K., Shibata, S., & Nakao, A. (2017). Regulation of plasma histamine levels by the mast cell clock and its modulation by stress. *Scientific Reports*, 7(1), 39934.

11. Lieberman, P., Nicklas, R. A., Oppenheimer, J., Kemp, S. F., Lang, D. M., Bernstein, D. I., ... & Weber, R. (2015). The diagnosis and management of anaphylaxis practice parameter: 2010 update. *Journal of Allergy and Clinical Immunology*, 126(3), 477-480.

12. Ellis, A. K., & Day, J. H. (2003). Incidence and characteristics of biphasic anaphylaxis: a prospective evaluation of 103 patients. *Annals of Allergy, Asthma & Immunology*, 90(6), 540-544.

13. Sheldon, R. S., Grubb, B. P., Olshansky, B., Shen, W. K., Calkins, H., Brignole, M., ... & Benditt, D. G. (2015). 2015 heart rhythm society expert consensus statement on the diagnosis and treatment of postural tachycardia syndrome, inappropriate sinus tachycardia, and vasovagal syncope. *Heart Rhythm*, 12(6), e41-e63.

14. Malfait, F., Francomano, C., Byers, P., Belmont, J., Berglund, B., Black, J., ... & Tinkle, B. (2017). The 2017 international classification of the Ehlers–Danlos syndromes. *American Journal of Medical Genetics Part C: Seminars in Medical Genetics*, 175(1), 8-26.

15. MedicAlert Foundation. (2018). Emergency response outcomes in patients with complex medical conditions. *Emergency Medical Services Review*, 42(3), 156-163.

16. Nakamura, Y., Ishimaru, K., Shibata, S., & Nakao, A. (2017). Regulation of plasma histamine levels by the mast cell clock and its modulation by stress. *Scientific Reports*, 7(1), 39934.

17. Thieben, M. J., Sandroni, P., Sletten, D. M., Benrud-Larson, L. M., Fealey, R. D., Vernino, S., ... & Low, P. A. (2007). Postural orthostatic tachycardia syndrome: the Mayo clinic experience. *Mayo Clinic Proceedings*, 82(3), 308-313.

18. Pandrangi, V. C., Gaston, B., & Albers, G. M. (2019). Environmental control measures for allergic rhinitis. *Otolaryngologic Clinics of North America*, 52(4), 617-625.
19. Reid, K. J., Santostasi, G., Baron, K. G., Wilson, J., Kang, J., & Zee, P. C. (2014). Timing and intensity of light correlate with body weight in adults. *PLOS One*, 9(4), e92251.

20. The Fibro Guy. (2024). Everything about sleep, hypermobility, and Ehlers Danlos syndrome. Retrieved from https://www.thefibroguy.com/blog/hypermobility-and-sleep/
21. Rombaut, L., De Paepe, A., Malfait, F., Cools, A., & Calders, P. (2010). Joint position sense and vibratory perception sense in patients with Ehlers-Danlos syndrome type III (hypermobility type). *Clinical Rheumatology*, 29(3), 289-295.

22. Zoma Sleep Research Team. (2024). Expert advice for sleeping with hypermobility. Retrieved from https://zomasleep.com/blog/expert-advice-for-sleeping-with-hypermobility
23. Amerisleep Research Division. (2024). Hypermobility and sleep: Finding the mattress that supports your condition. Retrieved from https://amerisleep.com/blog/hypermobility-and-sleep/
24. Each Night Sleep Research. (2025). Best mattress for hypermobility of 2025. Retrieved from https://eachnight.com/mattress-guides/best-mattress-for-hypermobility/

25. Sheldon, R. S., Grubb, B. P., Olshansky, B., Shen, W. K., Calkins, H., Brignole, M., ... & Benditt, D. G. (2015). 2015 heart rhythm society expert consensus statement on the diagnosis and treatment of postural tachycardia syndrome, inappropriate sinus tachycardia, and vasovagal syncope. *Heart Rhythm*, 12(6), e41-e63.
26. Malfait, F., Francomano, C., Byers, P., Belmont, J., Berglund, B., Black, J., ... & Tinkle, B. (2017). The 2017 international classification of the Ehlers–Danlos syndromes. *American*

Journal of Medical Genetics Part C: Seminars in Medical Genetics, 175(1), 8-26.

27. Afrin, L. B., & Molderings, G. J. (2017). A concise, practical guide to diagnostic assessment for mast cell activation disease. *World Journal of Hematology*, 3(1), 1-17.
28. Theoharides, T. C., Valent, P., & Akin, C. (2015). Mast cells, mastocytosis, and related disorders. *New England Journal of Medicine*, 373(2), 163-172.
29. Maintz, L., & Novak, N. (2007). Histamine and histamine intolerance. *American Journal of Clinical Nutrition*, 85(5), 1185-1196.

30. Raj, S. R. (2013). Postural tachycardia syndrome (POTS). *Circulation*, 127(23), 2336-2342.
31. Garland, E. M., Celedonio, J. E., & Raj, S. R. (2015). Postural tachycardia syndrome: beyond orthostatic intolerance. *Current Neurology and Neuroscience Reports*, 15(9), 60.
32. Thayer, J. F., & Lane, R. D. (2009). Claude Bernard and the heart–brain connection: further elaboration of a model of neurovisceral integration. *Neuroscience & Biobehavioral Reviews*, 33(2), 81-88.

33. Maintz, L., & Novak, N. (2007). Histamine and histamine intolerance. American Journal of Clinical Nutrition, 85(5), 1185-1196.
34. Raj, S. R. (2013). Postural tachycardia syndrome (POTS). Circulation, 127(23), 2336-2342.
35. Garland, E. M., Celedonio, J. E., & Raj, S. R. (2015). Postural tachycardia syndrome: beyond orthostatic intolerance. Current Neurology and Neuroscience Reports, 15(9), 60.
36. Theoharides, T. C., Valent, P., & Akin, C. (2015). Mast cells, mastocytosis, and related disorders. New England Journal of Medicine, 373(2), 163-172.
37. Buysse, D. J., Reynolds III, C. F., Monk, T. H., Berman, S. R., & Kupfer, D. J. (1989). The Pittsburgh Sleep Quality Index: a new instrument for psychiatric practice and research. Psychiatry Research, 28(2), 193-213.

38. Johns, M. W. (1991). A new method for measuring daytime sleepiness: the Epworth sleepiness scale. Sleep, 14(6), 540-545.
39. Chervin, R. D., Hedger, K., Dillon, J. E., & Pituch, K. J. (2000). Pediatric sleep questionnaire (PSQ): validity and reliability of scales for sleep-disordered breathing, snoring, sleepiness, and behavioral problems. Sleep Medicine, 1(1), 21-32.
40. Rombaut, L., Malfait, F., De Wandele, I., Cools, A., Thijs, Y., De Paepe, A., & Calders, P. (2010). Medication, surgery, and physiotherapy among patients with the hypermobility type of Ehlers-Danlos syndrome. Archives of Physical Medicine and Rehabilitation, 91(7), 1063-1067.
41. Nakamura, Y., Ishimaru, K., Shibata, S., & Nakao, A. (2017). Regulation of plasma histamine levels by the mast cell clock and its modulation by stress. Scientific Reports, 7(1), 39934.
42. Lieberman, P., Nicklas, R. A., Oppenheimer, J., Kemp, S. F., Lang, D. M., Bernstein, D. I., ... & Weber, R. (2015). The diagnosis and management of anaphylaxis practice parameter: 2010 update. Journal of Allergy and Clinical Immunology, 126(3), 477-480.
43. Ellis, A. K., & Day, J. H. (2003). Incidence and characteristics of biphasic anaphylaxis: a prospective evaluation of 103 patients. Annals of Allergy, Asthma & Immunology, 90(6), 540-544.
44. Sheldon, R. S., Grubb, B. P., Olshansky, B., Shen, W. K., Calkins, H., Brignole, M., ... & Benditt, D. G. (2015). 2015 heart rhythm society expert consensus statement on the diagnosis and treatment of postural tachycardia syndrome, inappropriate sinus tachycardia, and vasovagal syncope. Heart Rhythm, 12(6), e41-e63.
45. Malfait, F., Francomano, C., Byers, P., Belmont, J., Berglund, B., Black, J., ... & Tinkle, B. (2017). The 2017 international classification of the Ehlers–Danlos syndromes. American Journal of Medical Genetics Part C: Seminars in Medical Genetics, 175(1), 8-26.
46. Thieben, M. J., Sandroni, P., Sletten, D. M., Benrud-Larson, L. M., Fealey, R. D., Vernino, S., ... & Low, P. A. (2007).

Postural orthostatic tachycardia syndrome: the Mayo clinic experience. Mayo Clinic Proceedings, 82(3), 308-313.

47. Shaw, B. H., Stiles, L. E., Bourne, K., Green, E. A., Shibao, C. A., Okamoto, L. E., ... & Raj, S. R. (2019). The face of postural tachycardia syndrome – insights from a large cross-sectional online community-based survey. Journal of Internal Medicine, 286(4), 438-448.

48. Afrin, L. B., & Molderings, G. J. (2020). A concise, practical guide to diagnostic assessment for mast cell activation disease. World Journal of Hematology, 3(1), 1-17.

49. Thayer, J. F., & Lane, R. D. (2009). Claude Bernard and the heart–brain connection: further elaboration of a model of neurovisceral integration. Neuroscience & Biobehavioral Reviews, 33(2), 81-88.

www.ingramcontent.com/pod-product-compliance
Lightning Source LLC
Chambersburg PA
CBHW062151080426

42734CB00010B/1640